EAT YOUR WAY TO
SEXY

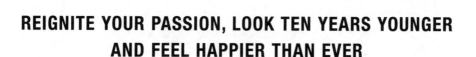

START LOSING WEIGHT IN JUST 7 DAYS!

REIGNITE YOUR PASSION, LOOK TEN YEARS YOUNGER
AND FEEL HAPPIER THAN EVER

ELIZABETH SOMER, MA, RD

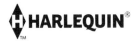

EAT YOUR WAY TO SEXY
ISBN-13: 978-0-373-89253-2
© 2012 by Elizabeth Somer

The nutritional and health advice presented in this book is based on an in-depth review of the current scientific literature. It is intended only as an informative resource guide to help you make informed decisions; it is not meant to replace the advice of a physician or to serve as a guide to self-treatment. Always seek competent medical help for any health condition or if there is any question about the appropriateness of a procedure or health recommendation.

A full list of references used in the writing of this book can be found at www.elizabethsomer.com.

Somer, Elizabeth.
    Eat your way to sexy / Elizabeth Somer.
        p. cm.
    ISBN 978-0-373-89253-2 (pbk.)
    1. Sexual health. 2. Women–Health and hygiene. 3. Women–Nutrition. I. Title.
    RG121.S667 2011
    613.9'54–dc22
                                2011011964

www.Harlequin.com
Printed in USA.

To Ward,
who makes me feel sexy
all the time

Also by Elizabeth Somer:

Eat Your Way to Happiness

• • •

Age-Proof Your Body

• • •

10 Habits that Mess Up a Woman's Diet

• • •

The Origin Diet

• • •

The Food & Mood Cookbook

• • •

Nutrition for a Healthy Pregnancy

• • •

Food & Mood

• • •

Nutrition for Women

• • •

The Essential Guide to Vitamins and Minerals

• • •

The Nutrition Desk Reference (coauthor)

CONTENTS

INTRODUCTION

What does sexy feel like? Take a moment, sit back, close your eyes and imagine what it is like to feel strong, attractive and sensual. To strut into a room confident, knowing you turn heads. Just for a moment, connect with the *You* that feels the most desirous, passionate, alive.

For a woman, part of that image might be wearing a pair of cute black high-heel stilettos, some lacy underthing from Victoria's Secret, or being ogled by the right bad boy. For a man, it might be wearing a tailored suit, walking a certain strut, driving a sports car or ogling the right cleavage. But I want you to go deeper than that. What are the feelings, attitudes, emotions that enticed you to put on the high heels or walk the walk in the first place? What does sexy feel like deep down inside? What fuels that passion?

I'm guessing that you'll find at the core of your sexy self a wellspring of positive feelings. You will find confidence, vitality and authenticity. You will find unlimited energy, aliveness and gusto. You even might find playfulness, youthfulness or a natural feeling of freedom. In short, when you are feeling genuinely comfortable in your own skin, happy, excited about life, and have the energy to be adventurous, it is then that you are likely to also feel your sexiest.

Sexy is far more than just a passing mood. It's not about wearing an expensive outfit or driving a racy car (although that's fun, too!). It is how you feel, how you act, how you look, how you live. The added benefit is that confidence and joy attract people to you. It brings out the sexy in others, too!

Circuitry and Circulation

Inside that sexy self, there is a whole lot of circuitry and circulation going on. For you to feel really sultry, powerful, alive requires a fine-tuned brain that sends messages quickly and freely, a healthy heart that pumps blood efficiently and easily, and clear and elastic blood vessels that effortlessly move blood and oxygen throughout your body, from head to sex organs. The better that circuitry and circulation work, the more energetic you feel and the better lover you will be. The building blocks and assembly-line workers for those well-revved systems come directly and only from your diet.

The relationship between what you eat and your sex life is like the fuel you put into a car. You wouldn't dream of packing the gas tank with sawdust, then expect the car to run at tip-top speed. Hey, you're lucky if it runs at all! It's exactly the same with your body. Pump the nutritional equivalent of sawdust into your body and you are more likely to feel like a jalopy than a race car. Put high-octane foods into that system, rev it up with a bit of exercise and you will pump up your thrill quotient and reconnect with the Maserati within. The thrust, if you will, is that nutritional deficiencies and/or excesses sap you mentally, physically and emotionally...and that saps mojo.

I see people all the time who are in poor health. They don't even know it. They aren't glaringly sick, but their circuitry and circulation are faulty all the same. They are tired, cranky, overweight, stressed out or feel emotionally drained. Their sex lives are unsatisfying, or sometimes nonexistent. Maybe the man can't get it up or the woman isn't interested. Their hair might be limp or their complexions pale. Some are on medications, others look older than their years. Their health problems have become their prisons. Most of them have no idea that their lives—in and out of the bedroom—could be so much easier, vital, energetic, radiant. I'm sure you see them, too. Perhaps you've been there, done that.

Well, don't. You can be so much *more*. Life has so much more to offer. All you have to do is make a few simple changes in how you nourish your body, mind and life to go beyond getting by and start living life to its fullest.

You Get One Chance at Sexy

You only get one body and one brain in this lifetime. What a shame to waste it! Instead, nourishing the body and mind is the direct route to sexy. Eat, move and live right and you will be amazed at how strong, confident, energized and sharp you are. At any age, you'll find that *It* in you, that mysterious quality that goes beyond just sex appeal. It's that quality that turns us on, that attracts people to us. It's radiance. It's that certain Something. You can have It when you take care of that wonderful body and brain of yours.

A perfect example is Laura, a 45-year-old schoolteacher I counseled in San Diego. At her first visit, she explained, "My husband and I had a great sex life until the kids were born. I let myself go after that. Now I'm tired all the time. I take care of babies, clean the house, work full time. I don't even have the energy to put on a dress, let alone frolic in the bedroom." Laura made all kinds of excuses as to why she deserved to be exhausted. She told me that she was juggling family and work, she was getting older, everyone around her was tired so why shouldn't she be, too? I didn't believe a word of it.

We all deserve to feel good. In fact, we deserve to feel great. Life is just too short and too wonderful to let it pass by unappreciated and unexplored. The catch is that feeling great doesn't just descend on us like a silky cloak. Ya gotta work at it, baby!

That's why I ignored Laura's excuses and, instead, asked her to give me a rundown on her diet. That diet explained volumes. Laura was working at it, but she was working at feeling awful, not great. She skipped meals, grabbed junk on the go, snacked on salty chips, ate late and often drank a tad too much wine in the evening. She also had shelved exercise. I asked her to make a few changes in what and when she ate (and emphasized that these changes would benefit her husband and kids, too) and had her promise to walk the dog every night to gradually add more activity back into her life.

> 66 *You can't separate what you eat and your lifestyle from your confidence, vibrancy or sexiness.* 99

Within a few weeks, Laura was back for her last session with a big smile on her face, a new haircut and wearing a cute sundress. "I don't know what has come over us, but my husband and I both have more energy, even after the kids are in bed. We put on a CD last night, lit a few candles and danced! I won't go into what followed in the bedroom!" she blushed.

You can't separate what you eat and your lifestyle from your confidence, vibrancy or sexiness. What you eat, how much you move, and how you choose to live affect your attitudes, thinking, emotions and physical health. You are one big package. You choose how sexy you are by the foods you choose to eat. Eat junk and you'll feel like junk. Eat well and your body will repay you a thousandfold with abundant energy, a sharper mind, a fit body and a lustier life. You, and only you, control your destiny to be well or sick. It's up to you. I hope you choose well.

DO YOU NEED SOME *mojo maintenance?*

If you answer "no" to any or all of these questions, you might be in need of a little mojo maintenance from the S-Ex-Y Diet and Fitness Program.

1. Do you feel strong and capable every day?

2. Are you very happy most of the time?

3. Are your memory, concentration and recall as good as they were years ago?

4. Would you rate your energy level—on a scale of 1 to 10—as 8 or above, with 10 being unlimited energy throughout the day?

5. Do you feel sexy and attractive most of the time?

6. Do people frequently comment that you look much younger than your years?

7. Do you have a strong, supportive circle of close friends and family that you connect with on a regular basis?

8. Are you at a weight that makes you feel vibrant, alive and proud?

9. Do you frequently get excited about and are ready to try new things?

10. Do you sleep soundly and wake up refreshed and energized?

11. Do you remain calm during stress and reduce daily tensions by exercising, meditating or other healthful habits, not with alcohol or drugs?

12. Can you run across the street to make the bus or bound up a flight of stairs without huffing and puffing?

13. Do you smile and laugh more nowadays than ever before?

14. Do you take few or no prescription medications?

15. Are you hopeful and excited about the future?

16. Are you as interested—or even more interested—in sex than you used to be?

17. Do you typically focus on your strengths and possibilities, not your weaknesses and problems?

18. Do you walk tall, with good posture and your chin up?

19. Are you satisfied with how your life is going?

20. Do you feel like these are your best years?

The S-Ex-Y Diet

I know how to revive or improve your sexy self. I know how you can put more spring in your step. I even know exactly what you need to improve your memory today and help prevent dementia down the road. I have studied the link between food and mood for decades. I've seen firsthand what a few changes can do for a person's mood, mind and memory. I've seen miracles happen over and over as people transform a good life into a great one by making a few changes in how they care for themselves.

I absolutely guarantee that if you follow the guidelines in the *Sensual Extraordinary You Diet*—the S-Ex-Y Diet—you will be happier, leaner and sexier than you ever have been before. You also will look younger, feel friskier and think faster. You'll enjoy sex more, respond and perform better and find your sex life more satisfying. Better yet, your entire life will be better. That's what happens when you fuel the Maserati within.

The S-Ex-Y eating plan in the following pages focuses on authentic foods, and includes simple guidelines for the Ménage à Trois breakfast, the G-Spot and Quickie snacks, the Twosome Lunch, and the Antioxidant Orgy. You'll learn about the wealth of foods in this plan that are "brain candy" for revving the mind at any age. You'll get a fatigue-busting makeover guaranteed to improve your energy level all day long and well into the night. If losing a few pounds makes you feel sexier, then the 12 super-sexy, foolproof tricks for permanent weight loss are right up your alley. You'll also learn how to tweak the S-Ex-Y Diet to nourish your skin so that you look up to 15 years younger. Herbs, spices and supplements that give an extra boost to the Diet will provide that competitive edge and turn a lagging mojo into a lusty one.

It's no secret that better health translates into a better sex life, with healthy people being the ones most likely to have sex and enjoy it the most. But I want more for you than that. It's not just about having sex and enjoying it, which is great in and of itself. It's about feeling alive, vibrant, confident, passionate. It's about saying "YES!" to life, in and out of the bedroom. I promise you can get there if you follow the suggestions in the following pages.

—Elizabeth Somer, MA, RD

part ONE

1.

ARE YOU IN
the mood?

THE PROMISE

Within **ONE WEEK** of making these changes, you will

✓ Notice improvements in your energy level.

In **ONE MONTH**, you will

✓ Be happier, more calm, more confident.

✓ Feel a bit friskier.

✓ Have more consistent energy throughout the day.

✓ Notice that people are commenting on the positive changes in your looks, energy, thinking and/or mood.

In **ONE YEAR**, you will

✓ Lose up to 50 pounds.

✓ If you have been on antidepressants, be on less or none.

✓ Be more sexually responsive and enjoy sex more.

✓ Be at an all-time high for happiness and satisfaction.

Carla had struggled with depression and a steady weight gain for five years, until she turned around her mood and waistline in a blink-of-an-eye "aha" moment.

After trying to get a grip on her life for several years, she went to a psychiatrist, who let her vent about frustrations and lack of energy. The doctor listened while Carla whined about her weight and how the sizzle had drained out of her love life. They both agreed that there didn't appear to be any major issues to explain the general funk. The psychiatrist suggested that Carla make some changes in her diet and lifestyle, maybe do some volunteer work, join the gym, talk to a dietitian. They brainstormed several options. Then, if all else failed, she'd prescribe a mild antidepressant.

That's how Carla ended up in my office. I was one of her homework assignments—see a dietitian, when that flops—which, of course, she assumed it would—then go back to the psychiatrist for medication. But, like so many best-laid plans, Carla's life was about to take a 180-degree turn.

A brief review of what she was eating made it crystal clear why she felt so bad and had gained 20 pounds. I concluded, "You're eating junk. No wonder you feel like junk." Carla looked me straight in the eye and I could tell a light had gone on in her mind.

"It was one of those 'aha' moments for me. The statement was so simple, yet it really hit home," says Carla. "I realized that since the baby was born, I'd fallen into this time mantra, telling myself over and over again that I didn't have enough time to work out, plan elaborate dinners or even bother with my weight or my looks. I was in the habit of grabbing quick-fix foods, like granola bars, chips or bean burritos from a taco stand on my way to work. I still made dinner most nights, but I'd cut corners there, too. I was addicted to Marie Callender's frozen entrées and more than once the family ate boxed mac and cheese for dinner. Yet I told myself I was eating pretty good. Hey, my eating habits were no worse than anyone else's! I knew my food choices had contributed to the weight gain, but it never dawned on me that my slow but steady diet demise paralleled my slide into fatigue and depression."

Carla is not alone. In fact, odds are you probably are just like her. Only one in every 100 people in this country meet even minimum standards of a balanced diet. I'm not talking optimal here. Just minimum!

The U.S. Department of Agriculture (USDA) developed a questionnaire to assess people's eating habits. It's called the Healthy Eating Index and it divides the diet into 10 categories, such as the amount of bad fat you eat, the number of servings of fruits and the amount of vegetables in the diet. A diet is ranked from 0 to 10 in each category. Eat the optimal amount of fruits, for example, and you'll score a ten in that category. Score perfectly in all 10 categories and you get 100%.

Few people come close to a passing grade on the Healthy Eating Index. Americans consistently average a score of 52 on the scale of 0 to 100. In other words, we flunk eating. If our kids came home with a score like that on a math test, we'd ground them and hire tutors. Yet most people when asked how they rate their eating habits, answer that they think they do "Not great, but pretty well." Virtually all of them are delusional!

Have You Lost That Lovin' Feeling?

As our eating habits took a nosedive in the past few decades, the rates of depression skyrocketed.

Today, depression is a leading cause of disability, second only to high blood pressure. Almost 15 million Americans are battling serious depression. Another 3.3 million hide under the sad umbrella most of the time. About 7 out of 10 Americans are overweight, which increases their risk for depression. (As people lose weight, their mood improves.) Not only does depression undermine a person's enjoyment of life, but it increases the risk fourfold for other health problems, such as heart disease. It also is the fast track to Frumpville, since 7 out of 10 people battling the blues say they lost their mojo somewhere down the road. In short, you can't get to sexy if you are chained to the blues wagon.

Most people turn to medication first to solve the problem. Antidepressants like Prozac are prescribed more often than any other pill besides the birth control pill. I am not saying there isn't a place for medication when you're trying to "fix" depression, but drugs are not the Holy Grail of treatment, either. For one thing, up to 40% of people don't respond to these medications and even those who do, report the drugs don't erase the problem. Meds might make some people feel closer to normal or at least help them blunt the pain. But those drugs also can destroy sex drive, cloud thinking and kick self-confidence in the butt, which then undermines mood, leading to an even lower sex drive. Medication also comes with a few other nasty side effects, including fatigue, weight gain (up to 9 pounds a month!) and impotence. I'm not sure what is worse—the bad mood or the side effects from the drugs to treat it!

MOVIES TO GET YOU
in the mood

1. **9½ Weeks**
   (Mickey Rourke, Kim Basinger, 1986)

2. **Body Heat**
   (William Hurt, Kathleen Turner, 1998)

3. **The Postman Always Rings Twice**
   (Jack Nicholson, Jessica Lange, 1981)

4. **The Lover**
   (Jane March, Tony Leung Ka Fai, 1992)

5. **Damage**
   (Jeremy Irons, Juliette Binoche, 1992)

6. **The Bridges of Madison County**
   (Meryl Streep, Clint Eastwood, 1995)

7. **Bull Durham**
   (Susan Sarandon, Kevin Costner, 1988)

8. **Pretty Woman**
   (Julia Roberts, Richard Gere, 1990)

9. **Dirty Dancing**
   (Patrick Swayze, Jennifer Grey, 1987)

A Mood Makeover

Luckily, Carla's psychiatrist felt it was worth her trying some life changes before she started popping pills. It worked. Once Carla fueled her body with the foods it needed to run well, her weight started dropping, while her mood improved.

Like Carla, you can reclaim and sustain hope, joy, an upbeat attitude and a confident spirit by making a few simple adjustments to how you treat your body and your life...with not one single side effect other than improved energy, lower disease risk, a slimmer waistline and a return of that mojo!

Let's get this straight right now. This is important, so listen up. You were not designed to be tired, depressed or overweight. It is not one of our basic survival skills. None of those modern-day problems would have served our ancient ancestors well on the savannah a million years ago. Our species survived because our ancestors were mentally and physically strong. A tired, grumpy, fat caveman would not have outrun a saber-toothed tiger, or would have been left behind when the tribe moved on. (Who's got time to give Ukluk a pep talk when the Ice Age is coming?) Depression and obesity are results of civilization, not genes. They are not "normal." They are not instinct, destiny or inevitable.

You also were not designed to eat Pop-Tarts, Cheez Whiz, white bread, potato chips or soft drinks. In fact, most of the more than 30,000 items at your local grocery store never crossed the lips of any of our ancient ancestors, dating back millions of years. The Pilgrims would not recognize our modern excuse for food, either. Even a Civil War soldier would be amazed at what we are putting in our mouths. In short, our eating habits have changed astronomically in the past 100 years, yet we are genetically identical to our ancient ancestors who evolved and thrived for eons on diets composed of fruits, vegetables, root plants, wild grass seed, wild game, seafood, nuts and a bit of honey.

Processed foods—made with refined grains, added sugars, fat, salt, additives, colorants, stabilizers, preservatives and more—are as alien to your body as breathing carbon monoxide. Put junk into your body and guess what? You get fat, tired, obstinate, depressed, forgetful and cranky. And you end up with a team of physicians doing damage control.

That's what had happened to Carla. The general malaise that had taken over her life crept up slowly and steadily as she turned her back on the foods that sustain a happy, vibrant, sexy life. Instead, she wolfed down processed junk. Eat junk and you will feel, look and act like junk.

But—and here's the great part!—eat well and, I promise, like Carla, it will turn your life around. You'll be happier, leaner, more energetic, and you will feel sexier!!! The better you eat, the healthier and more vibrant you are. The healthier you are, the sexier you feel.

Carla followed the diet advice I gave her that day. She slowly adopted the six rules from the S-Ex-Y Diet (the _S_ensual _Ex_traordinary _Y_ou Diet) and within six weeks, she had dropped 12 of the 20 pounds she wanted to lose, had canceled the follow-up appointment with the doctor ("Who needs drugs when you can feel this good with food?") and even her coworkers noticed her newfound energy.

Your Brain on Happiness

> **66** *It isn't what you have, or who you are, or where you are, or what you are doing that makes you happy or unhappy. It is what you think about.* **99**
> —George Sheehan, MD

Finding joy means opening yourself to it. Happiness is a skill you learn and nurture. A great place to start is with how you nourish yourself and, therefore, that joy.

It really is simple. People who eat right are the happiest. People who eat junk are more prone to sadness, and have the highest rates of depression. The worse their food choices, the worse they feel. As soon as they make changes in their diets, they start feeling better. The more changes they make, the better they feel. They also lose weight, lower their risk for all age-related diseases, such as heart disease, and even report improvements in their sex lives! No matter who you are—man, woman, young, old, black, brown, yellow, white or purple, and in every country—you will experience the same benefits.

Adopting the S-Ex-Y Diet also starts a spiral that becomes a self-perpetuating stream of bliss. People who turn the grump ship around with a few adjustments to their diets find they attract more happiness. They have the energy to be generous and less self-focused, so they enrich the lives of those around them. People are drawn to them and feel better when they are, like moths to a flame. It's like the old saying, "You catch more bees with honey than with vinegar." When you are happy and share that happiness, you get back happy a hundredfold!

I absolutely guarantee if you adopt the six guidelines of the diet, you will feel the best you have ever felt. I've seen it work over and over again for decades, just as it worked for Carla. The closer you stick to the plan and the longer you stick with it, the better you will feel, the better your mood and the more energy you will have to embrace life to its fullest. Just follow these six S-Ex-Y Diet guidelines:

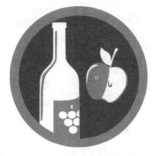

(1) Have an antioxidant orgy.

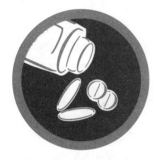

(6) Take the pill.

6

S-Ex-Y Diet
GUIDELINES

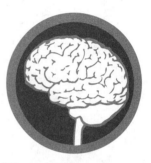

(2) Feed your #1 sex organ.

(5) Remember that
size matters.

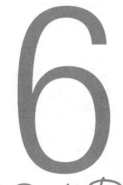

(4) Get wet and wild
at least twice a week.

(3) Give yourself some space.

I will discuss each of these guidelines in detail throughout the book. For now, it is enough to know the basics.

#1: Have an antioxidant orgy Load your plate with foods rich in antioxidants, such as colorful fruits and vegetables, legumes, herbs and spices, and red wine. Aim for at least nine servings a day. More is even better. These foods protect the brain from damage associated with memory loss and depression, and also boost the body's defenses against inflammation.

#2: Feed your #1 sex organ If risqué thoughts pop into your head when you hear the words sex organ, that's exactly where they should be, since your #1 sex organ is your brain! Here lies not only your favorite fantasies, but also a stew of mood and appetite chemicals, called neurotransmitters, that can be tweaked into submission if you eat the right foods at the right time and in the right amounts.

#3: Give yourself some space When you eat is as important as what you eat. The right spacing of meals and snacks boosts mood and energy. Also, one beverage and certain snacks (you'll read more later about the G-Spot snack and the Perfect Quickies), spaced throughout the day, can improve your mood, help you sleep and jump-start your thinking.

#4: Get wet and wild at least twice a week Some foods and their nutrients are so important that you need to include them at least a few times a week. In this batch is the omega-3 fat DHA found in fatty fish like salmon.

#5: Remember that size matters While I dare you to eat too many vegetables, limiting portions of other foods will make a huge difference when it comes to mood, mind, memory and, of course, your waistline.

#6: Take the pill No matter how well you eat, it is likely you will need a supplement or two to fill in the gaps on the days when you don't eat perfectly, as well as to give you that extra edge when it comes to feeling friskier, happier and more energetic.

That Loving Relationship

Every time you bite into an apple, take a forkful of mashed potatoes, or a gulp of orange juice, you embrace the most intimate relationship of your life.

> 66 *It's a very odd thing*
> *As old as can be*
> *That whatever Miss T eats*
> *Turns into Miss T.* 99
> —Walter de la Mare

You already know that food sustains you. It supplies the energy (in calories) you need to raise a finger, get yourself out of bed in the morning, keep your heart pumping, your hair growing and, if consumed in excess, your hips widening.

That is just the tip of the nutritional iceberg. Every bit of you comes from your diet. Every atom. Every molecule. Every single cell, tissue, organ, system is made entirely from what you have eaten and gulped in the past and are eating today. There is nowhere else, other than the oxygen you breathe, for your body to get its building blocks. The billions of cells in your body are made up of the fat you ate in a French fry or an almond, the protein that makes up your organs and tissues came from the Big Mac or the salmon steak you had yesterday, the calcium in your bones came from the glass of milk you drank last week, while the magnesium that regulates your stress hormones came from the spinach salad at lunch.

You probably know all this. Most people understand the intimate relationship between what they eat and their physical health. Eat too many Big Macs and you end up with clogged arteries and heart disease. Drink too little milk and someday you are likely to be a stooped, old lady (or man) with osteoporosis. It takes years for those physical symptoms to show up, but believe me, for most people, they will.

What you choose to eat today has a much more immediate impact on your mood. Literally, what you eat or don't eat for breakfast will have a subtle effect on how you feel and think midday. What you ate last week already is influencing how happy you are right now. The effects also are cumulative. Whether you are happy or sad, clearheaded or muddled, energized or barely dragging your "you know what" out of bed in the morning is a direct result of what you ate all month, all year and all your life. So stop blaming a crummy mood or a muddled mind on your genes. According to the National Institute on Aging, only 15–20% of aging is genetic; that means up to 85% is entirely up to you and the choices, including the food choices, you make!

There is a very good reason why your diet becomes your mood. The more than 100 billion cells in your brain are surrounded by a coating, called a membrane, that is made up of fats from the diet. Eat the right fats and those membranes are fluid and flexible, able to relay with ease messages from one brain cell to another. The brain cell receptors also run in tip-top condition. You think fast, remember well and have high levels of the feel-good chemicals, such as serotonin, in the brain. On the other hand, eat the wrong fats and those brain cell membranes are rigid, inflexible and less able to send messages. The receptors crumble and, as a result, you are moody, depressed and don't think clearly. Down the road, you are at high risk for dementia and even Alzheimer's disease. Those fatty brain cell membranes are protected from damage by the almost 1 million phytonutrients in foods, too.

What you eat also influences the ebb and flow of brain chemicals. Neurotransmitters—from serotonin, neuropeptide Y (NPY) and galanin to acetylcholine, the endorphins and more—regulate everything from emotions, moods and memories to your likes and dislikes, opinions and sense of humor. All those mood-regulating chemicals are made from components in your diet, and many also are turned on or off by what you choose to eat.

For example, serotonin likes carbohydrates. Eat an all-carb snack, and levels of this feel-good chemical (it's the neurotransmitter that many of the antidepressant medications raise) jump to attention. Other components of your diet, like vitamins and minerals, are assembly-line workers in the brain's production of cells, nerve chemicals and supporting structures. I could go on and on.

In short, our moods are not so much dependent on what happens *to* us as what happens *inside* us. Next time you find yourself blaming your spouse for putting you in a bad mood, think again. What you feed yourself is probably a far bigger reason for your gloomy mood.

The Authentic Lover

Now, let's take this one step further. Researchers studying the outside factors that influence happiness, such as money, work, where we live and what we own, have concluded that *the* most important thing we can do for our happiness quotient is to be part of loving, supportive, honest, nurturing relationships. Everything else pales in comparison to that one essential part of life. *(See Chapter 10.)*

What about the internal factors? Isn't supporting and nurturing a healthy relationship with the center of not just your life but your being—that would be

> **66** *Real food is more than just calories that get you through the day.* **99**

you—fundamental to happiness? And, since what you put in your mouth is the most intimate relationship you ever will have with yourself, it makes sense that true happiness begins with a supportive relationship with honest, authentic, real food.

Real food is more than just calories that get you through the day. Authentic food is packed with all the nutrient goodies your brain and body need to thrive, glow and work in perfect harmony. It's no surprise that researchers all over the world have found that the more authentic food people eat, the happier and lustier they are.

What is authentic food? It is food that is unprocessed, real, and comes with little packaging or few ingredients. It is food that grows on a plant or has fins or legs. It is colorful fruits, vegetables, whole grains, legumes, lean meats or seafood, low-fat milk products or foods made from these basic ingredients. It is foods our ancestors evolved on. Eat authentic and you will feel a whole lot closer to blissfully happy, healthy, strong, confident and...yes, sexy.

Authentic is where you start if you want to beat the blues. Focus on nourishing your mood with true, honest, authentic foods. Build a relationship with the real stuff, not the big-talking, B.S.ing, bad-boy foods. You want the apple, not the apple chips. The fresh spinach, not the frozen spinach in cream sauce. The steel-cut oats, not the maple-flavored instant oatmeal. The wild salmon, not the packaged bologna. The oven-baked yam, not the fast-food French fry.

How Much Loving Do You Need?

Ideally, every food that graces your lips should be authentic. But I'm also a realist and know that in this toxic environment, where every street has a fast-food restaurant, vending machines are bulging with candy and chips, and even department stores, gas stations and bookstores now have scone-pushing coffee shops, it is not likely that you are going to eat perfectly every day, no matter how determined you are to be happy, healthy and sexy.

So let's compromise. I'll give you a little wiggle room if you promise to eat mostly authentic foods. Your goal is to eat authentic 75% of the time. That means three out of every four bites—three-quarters of the plate—should be colorful fruits and vegetables, 100% whole grains, nuts, seeds, seafood, extra-lean meat and low- or nonfat milk products. You can lace that authentic diet with junk 25% of the time—a handful of chips here, a small piece of chocolate cake there. Of course, the more authentic foods you eat, the better your mood, the more likely you'll fit into that little black dress or studly suit and the sexier you'll feel, while the more you "fudge" on the junk, the more your mood and mojo will plummet. All the snacks, meals, recipes and menus in this book will follow this one rule—at least three-quarters of the foods will be mood-boosting, sexy-making, authentic foods.

Four Secrets to Eating Authentic

> **66** *It might feel good getting fat, but it feels even better being fit and sexy.* **99**

I know switching from Pop-Tarts to oatmeal in the morning may be a stretch for some people. But quit whining. You won't get any sympathy, since you are the one battling the blues, not me. If you really, really want to feel great, confident, happy and sexy, you have to put a little effort into the program. There are no free lunches, baby! Keep in mind: It might feel good *getting* fat, but it feels even better *being* fit and sexy.

Besides, those happy, sexy people out there didn't get that way eating chips and sitting on the couch watching reruns of *American Idol*. Anyone over the age of 30 who is happy, healthy, lean and sexy is working at it. Trust me.

Take, for example, Camille, who has lost 22 pounds after following my advice. "In the old days, you would have found junk foods in my kitchen. Not any more. At first it was a conscious effort and I still have to be mindful, particularly when eating out, but I eat mostly real foods now. In the past, every road trip included a fast-food meal. Now, when I make the six-hour drive to visit family, we bring a food stash with us, like almonds, fruit, low-fat cheese and whole-wheat bagels. Then we enjoy a nice break from the road at a rest stop. Elizabeth's book, *Eat Your Way to Happiness*, made me realize how much added sugar was in my diet, particularly foods that weren't even sweet—like salad dressing, ketchup, marinades, sauces. Cutting out the junk has made such a difference! The end result? I feel the best I've ever felt. I walk taller, feel fantastic and I get compliments all the time on how great I look. I don't mind that at all!"

I am well aware that it takes more time and discipline to plan meals, menus and snacks around authentic food than it does to take medication for depression. But the effort will repay you a thousandfold. For a little delayed gratification of saying "no" to a Quarter Pounder today, you will boost your mood, lose weight, have more energy, think more clearly, look younger and feel sexier tomorrow. You'll also live longer, which means more days of happy and sexy.

I'll even give you four secrets guaranteed to make switching to an authentic diet easier than ordering takeout.

Secret #1: Evict the junk. The more junk-food temptation you clear from the house, the easier it will be to stick with the plan. Remove the junk so it won't control your life.

Secret #2: Store the stash. Restock empty cupboards with authentic foods. The Authentic Shopping List on page 192 helps you get started.

Secret #3: Carry the goodies. Always bring authentic foods with you. You won't find mangos or baby carrots at a drive-through, so pack your lunch, snacks or nibbles when you are on the go.

Secret #4: Keep it simple. The biggest time-saver is making a weekly menu and shopping list. Plan and shop Sunday afternoon for the whole week. Organize the list by area in the grocery store to save more time. Cook in batches for multiple meals throughout the week. Use time-saving gadgets, such as a microwave, a food processor and a toaster oven. Use quick-fix items, like bagged lettuce, instant brown rice and frozen stir-fry veggies.

The G-Spot Stop

 Authentic foods are the foundation of the S-Ex-Y Diet and the surefire way to boost your mood. You can get an extra kick with a few tricks in my feel-great diet bag. One of them is including a G-Spot snack in the afternoon.

The *G* in G-Spot stands for grains. Whole grains. These are the carb-rich foods that give you an extra mood boost. If you are a carb craver, there could be a very good reason why those grains are so tempting.

Have you ever wondered why we turn to doughnuts, Ding Dongs and Doritos for solace when we are down in the dumps? Why not broccoli and wheat germ? There's a method to our moody madness and it starts at the very foundation of our being—our nerve cells. The carbs in sweets, chips or any grain tweak a bunch of body chemicals, especially the neurotransmitter serotonin, that regulate how we feel, act, and even what foods we crave.

From pasta to pie, carbs trigger the release of the hormone insulin from the pancreas, which, in turn, lowers blood levels of protein fragments, called amino acids. All except one—tryptophan, which just happens to be the building block for serotonin. Normally, tryptophan competes with other amino acids for entry into the brain, but with reduced competition, tryptophan has a clear shot through the blood-brain barrier. Once through the door, it is converted into serotonin, the feel-good neurotransmitter. Raise serotonin levels and you are happier, sleep better, feel sexier and more confident, and stop craving carbs.

> 66 *Serotonin is key to feeling motivated, having self-confidence and being enthusiastic about life.* 99

On the other hand, when serotonin levels drop, you feel blue, lose interest in life, are tired, and your sexy self is shelved. Serotonin is key to feeling motivated, having self-confidence and being enthusiastic about life. No wonder you crave carbs when you are cranky! Those cravings are an unconscious attempt to self-medicate, since the foods you crave are the very foods that will raise serotonin levels in the brain and de-funk your mood.

Sweet Sadness

Not all carbs are created equal. While a plate of pasta might calm you down, a sugar binge could leave you feeling blue and totally disinterested in sex. Depression and fatigue subside in some people when sugar (or caffeine) are removed from the diet. People first report improvements in energy level, then the depression lifts.

Even when sugar gives you a boost, it is only a temporary fix. In the long run, it could create a vicious cycle. Turn to candy to feel better and it might work in the short run, but the depression and fatigue return in no time. Back you go for more candy, and the spiral continues. As opposed to the temporary sugar high, eliminating sugar and caffeine from the diet, while including a G-Spot snack midafternoon, is a permanent solution.

G-Spot Boogie

The G-Spot snack is an all-carb minimeal designed to raise serotonin, while keeping blood sugar levels on an even keel. This is not permission to throw a one-person Cheetos party! You only need about 30 grams of carbs to get the serotonin boost and you must make sure there is little or no protein in the snack, since that would block tryptophan from getting into the brain. Those carbs should also come from whole grains, since they enter the bloodstream slowly to provide a slow, steady release of energy. About an ounce of whole grain supplies those 30 grams. Here are seven G-Spot snacks to get you through the week:

- 8 whole-wheat saltine crackers with 1 tablespoon fat-free cream cheese and 2 tablespoons mango chutney
- 6 ounces tabbouleh
- 1 small whole-grain tortilla with ½ sliced banana and 1 teaspoon honey
- 1 small apple and 3 graham crackers
- ⅓ cup mini shredded wheat mixed with 2 tablespoons dried tart cherries
- 1 whole-wheat pita bread toasted and cut into wedges. Dip in ⅓ cup salsa.
- 4 cups air-popped popcorn

It takes about half an hour for the carb to get from the mouth into the blood, and for tryptophan to squeeze through the blood-brain barrier into the brain. Plan that G-Spot snack about 30 minutes before you discuss a raise with your boss, confront your partner about an unpaid bill, tuck yourself into bed at night or expect your cravings for a cookie to begin, and by the time you walk through the door or hit the hay, you'll feel calmer, happier and more composed.

Wet, Wild and Perky

 Like soap-opera characters, dietary fat is either all good or all bad. Of the all-good fats, only one clearly boosts mood (and brainpower, but we'll get to that in Chapter 3). It's the omega-3 fat DHA (short for docohexaenoic acid, which is a mouthful, so let's stick to the DHA nickname).

Your brain is 60% fat and requires more DHA than any other tissue. As I mentioned before, each of the 100 billion brain cells packed in your cranium are encased in a fatty membrane that sends messages to other brain cells, eliminates toxins, absorbs oxygen and nutrients, and basically regulates what goes in and out of each of those cells. As we said earlier, the more fluid and flexible those membranes, the faster and more efficient your brain functions and the better your mood. The omega-3 fats, especially DHA, are the most fluid of all the fats and make the best brain-cell membranes.

Your body can't make this fat, so it is entirely dependent on your diet. It prefers these fats, but when you neglect to eat them, the brain turns elsewhere for its building blocks. More rigid fats are used instead. The end result? You are one cranky, depressed dummy.

You have almost a threefold higher chance of battling depression when your diet and brain are low in DHA. In fact, as DHA levels drop, so do brain cell receptors and levels of the feel-good brain chemical serotonin, leaving people grumpy, unmotivated, fatigued and downright depressed. As tissue levels of omega-3s drop, depression worsens. Of course, just the opposite is true, too. Around the world, the more fish (i.e., DHA) people eat, the more DHA is packed into brain cells and the lower the depression rates. Those eating the most fish have a 60-fold lower risk!!

The good news is this: Start caring for your brain by increasing your intake of this omega-3 fat and you jump-start your mood. There is a 50% reduction in depression in people who are the toughest to treat and even an improvement in well-being for those battling an everyday grump, just by adding omega-3s to the diet. A study from Greece determined that even one serving a week of salmon supplied enough DHA to reduce depression rates by 42%. The evidence is so strong, that the American Psychiatric Association recommends that these omega-3s be included with any treatment for depression.

> 66 . . . get wet and wild by eating fatty fish at least twice a week . . . 99

Live on the Wet and Wild Side

There are three omega-3 fats and they are not all created equal. The omega-3 in flaxseed or walnuts lowers heart disease risk, but has no proven benefits for mood. It is only the omega-3s in fatty fish, such as salmon, mackerel, herring or sardines, that boost mood and, of those, DHA is by far the biggest mood booster. These fish oils also reduce the risk for other brain disorders, from bipolar and anxiety disorders to aggression and possibly attention deficit. They might even enhance the effectiveness of antidepressant medications.

If you are prone to the blues and want to find yourself on the sunnier (and sexier) side of life, then get wet and wild by eating fatty fish at least twice a week, take a fish oil capsule that contains at least 1,000 milligrams of a combination of EPA and DHA, or include at least 220 milligrams of DHA from supplements or foods fortified with a vegetarian, algal DHA.

Nutrients That Spark a Good Mood

The S-Ex-Y Diet based on authentic food is not only loaded with healthy fats that build a happier brain, whole grains that raise levels of the feel-good chemicals and almost a million antioxidant-rich phytonutrients to protect brain tissue from damage, but it also guarantees that you'll get enough of the vitamins and minerals known to put you in the right mood for life and love.

All 40+ nutrients, as well as the fiber and phytonutrients in authentic foods, are like spark plugs, kick-starting and maintaining your mental, emotional and physical engines. Every nutrient plays a role in keeping you happy and ensuring that you remain energetic, disease-free and feeling sexy and alive. However, some nutrients are either a bit more important than others to your mood and sex life or have been more thoroughly researched. Here are the top 10 on the feel-great list and some of the foods in the S-Ex-Y Diet where you will get your fill:

1. Folate (spinach, chard, legumes, oranges, whole grains)
2. Vitamin B_{12} (chicken breast, salmon, fortified soymilk, yogurt)
3. Vitamin B_6 (seafood, low-fat milk, whole grains, avocados, bananas)
4. Magnesium (nuts, leafy greens, wheat germ, black beans)
5. Selenium (Brazil nuts, lean meat, kidney beans, vegetables grown in selenium-rich soil)
6. Vitamin D (fatty fish, fortified milk, soymilk, orange juice)
7. Vitamin E (nuts, seeds, avocado, mango, beet greens, kale, soybeans)
8. Vitamin C (citrus fruits, red bell peppers, fresh currants, broccoli, strawberries, kiwi)
9. Zinc (seafood, especially oysters; whole grains; legumes; plain yogurt; extra-lean meat)
10. Calcium (low- or nonfat milk or yogurt, dark green leafy vegetables, bones in canned fish, low-fat cheese, calcium-fortified soymilk, orange juice)

All these foods contribute to depression when you eat too little of them and boost mood when you get enough. For example, include enough folate-rich foods in your diet and your risk for depression drops like a rock. Too little folate and . . . oops, rates

I'M FEELING
sexy tricks

While switching to an authentic diet, you can put yourself on the fast-track to sexy with a few added tricks, such as:

Get Flirty: Add a little mischief to your mood to destress and feel good. A study from the University of Washington found that flirting in the workplace helps people feel happier, too. Flirting, when appropriate, also raises levels of the "love hormone," called oxytocin.

Act Up, Just a Little: A little mischief can go a long way to spicing up your love life. The touch of adrenalin is arousing, making you feel "more alive." I'm not talking about anything illegal or dangerous here. No shoplifting or weapons, please! Instead, try something out of the ordinary, spontaneous, exciting. Go to the airport with a backpack and take an unplanned flight to somewhere exotic. Or, play hooky from work and go for a hike in the woods or along the beach. Make out with your lover in public.

Strip: OK. Some of you might not be too excited about taking off all your clothes and parading around the house like a runway model. But letting your skin breathe without the confines of clothing is good for the body and soul. If this is just too much to ask, then try wearing all-natural fibers, such as cotton that breathes and is made with few or no chemicals.

Think Naughty: Dump the negative thoughts and let a little fantasy run wild in your head once in a while. Daydream a romantic or sexy encounter. Pick up a romance novel or watch a lusty movie (see page 6 for suggestions).

Dunk: Jump in a hot tub with a glass of bubbly. Then, talk dirty. Wink. Tell sexy stories.

Rub It In: Get a massage before a hot date. It will get you in touch with your body, relax you and help set the mood.

of depression skyrocket and you are less responsive to anti-depressant medications. Folate works with vitamins B_{12} and B_6 to lower a compound called homocysteine in the blood, which otherwise damages arteries and contributes to inflammation associated with depression. B_6 also is an assembly-line worker in the production of serotonin. *(See Chapter 3 for more on inflammation.)*

Magnesium and mood are a catch-22. The more depressed and stressed you are, the more magnesium you lose in your urine. As magnesium levels drop, you become more depressed and stressed. (Note: Men are also more prone to premature ejaculation when magnesium levels are low.) Calcium, along with magnesium, might also boost mood by altering hormone levels, aiding in nerve transmission or relaxation of muscles and helping regulate thyroid function.

One of the main reasons people are most prone to depression during the winter months is because they don't get enough sunlight, which is essential for the body to make vitamin D. No sunlight, no vitamin D. No vitamin D, no happy mood. Even interest in sex dwindles. Interestingly, fertility rates get a shot in the arm when men increase their intake of vitamin D. (Could it be because the vitamin puts them in a friskier mood?)

Blood levels should be between 50 to 80 ng/mL. Jeanette, a nurse in Oregon, found that her levels were only 5. "No wonder I was so down in the dumps during the winter," she said. "The doctor put me on 50,000 units a week until the levels approached the healthy range, then I dropped down to a maintenance dose of 5,000 units. It's like a dark cloud has lifted off my shoulders. I feel great now!"

The antioxidants, such as vitamins E and C, protect delicate brain tissue from damage associated with depression. Vitamin E, along with zinc, also has a nice little effect on a man's sperm, making them healthier and more active.

Get In The Mood, Now!

You have no excuse. There is something you can do, starting today, to get out of a funk, improve your enjoyment of life, enhance your self-confidence and give your sexier side a kick in the butt! Eat authentic 75% of the time, include a G-Spot snack midday, and eat no fewer than two servings a week of fatty fish or at least 220 milligrams of the omega-3 fat DHA every day. It works. I promise!

2

CAN YOU
get it up?

THE PROMISE

Within **ONE WEEK** of making these changes, you will

✓ Notice improvements in your energy level.

In **ONE MONTH**, you will

✓ Think more clearly.
✓ Have more consistent energy throughout the day.
✓ Notice a lessening of midday food cravings.
✓ Sleep more soundly.
✓ Awake more refreshed.

In **ONE YEAR**, you will

✓ Lose 20 pounds or more.
✓ Maintain a consistently high energy level throughout the day.
✓ Have more energy reserves in the evening for romance.

Terry, a home-health nurse, knew her energy slump had gone too far when, while unloading the groceries, she stored the milk in the cupboard and tossed the canned beans in the freezer. "That really scared me. All I could think of was, if I was that tuned-out on simple tasks, what mistakes was I making with my patients, my kids and the rest of my life?!"

She described her fatigue to her doctor, explaining that she often was cranky and snapped at both her husband and her kids, seldom had the energy to exercise and found herself dragging through the day, shuffling from one cup of coffee to the next. She was so exhausted at night that she often woke the next morning unable to recall the TV show she'd watched the night before. Her bloodwork came back normal, and the doctor concluded that she was doing too much for a woman her age. "On the drive home from the doctor's office, I was fuming. My age? My age! Since when is 37 old? I've always had boundless energy, and never settled for anything short of the best. Now I was so tired that my whole life was mediocre. Right then and there I decided it was time to get my groove back!"

Terry was ready for a fatigue-busting makeover, starting with her diet, which needed a total overhaul. She would find that eating to fuel her energy from morning to night would bring back that "boundless energy."

You Must be Up to be Sexy

Our energy level shapes who we are and how our lives unfold. It is the underlying source of passion, stamina, ambition, vitality, curiosity, joy and desire.

> 66 *Energy is eternal delight.* 99
> —William Blake

Abundant energy encourages openness to new things, playfulness, willingness to change. It's the "zing" in our lives, the "spark" in our humor and the "spring" in our step. Without abundant energy we are too pooped to pucker.

Energetic people typically have self-confidence and, yes, irresistible sexuality. When you are upbeat, energetic and vibrant, you are physically more attractive and feel better about yourself. In other words, you feel sexier. More energy means you radiate self-assurance, and those vibes make people want to share your enthusiasm. So why do one in four Americans put up with a lack of "oomph" so debilitating that it interferes with their sex lives? Especially since making just a few changes in how you fuel your body can have such fabulous results!

Why is nutrition critical to your energy and sexuality? Because, just as a flower droops when you don't fertilize and water it, so will your body. Each of the trillions of cells in your body, from brain to toes, is built and functions based on the vitamins, minerals, proteins, carbs, antioxidants and more that come from the diet. That's where the S-Ex-Y Diet comes in. It supplies all the nutrients in the right ratios and amounts, which in turn restores hormone balance, jump-starts metabolism, improves blood flow and revs energy. It keeps you primed for peak performance all day long.

It turns out that Terry was experiencing an energy crisis, fueled by her bad food choices. Her family, work and other relationships were front and center in her life, but she had overlooked the most important relationship of all—the one with herself. The good news is that her energy-draining diet habits gave us lots of room for improvement in getting back her mojo.

Here's an hour-by-hour account of how Terry ate to regain her energy, life and sexy self.

TERRY'S FATIGUE BUSTING
makeover

BEFORE	AFTER
7:00 a.m. Wake up, coffee	7:00 a.m. Wake up, write 5 reasons why I deserve to be energized. Coffee, shower/dress, make lunches
8:00 a.m. Feed kids, shower/dress, coffee	8:00 a.m. Feed kids and self (cereal, milk, fruit)
8:20 a.m. Leave for work	8:20 a.m. Leave for work w/lunch
10:30 a.m. Coffee	10:30 a.m. Snack: Yogurt, nuts, orange, water
1:00 p.m. Lunch at the drive-through, coffee, large cola	1:00 p.m. Exercise for 15 minutes. Lunch: Turkey sandwich on whole wheat, spinach salad w/oranges, carton of low-fat milk. Take multivitamin
4:00 p.m. Snack: Large coffee and muffin	4:30 p.m. Snack: String cheese, whole-grain crackers, apple, water
6:30 p.m. Glass of wine, grazing while heating frozen dinners in microwave	7:00 p.m. Dinner: Salmon, broccoli, salad, brown rice, red wine. Take calcium & DHA supplement
7:00 p.m. 2nd glass of wine with dinner	7:45 p.m. Brisk walk or stationary bike—30 minutes
9:30 p.m. Snack: Ice cream sundae, cookies, chips	9:30 p.m. Finish a project, make lunches
10:00 p.m. Crash in front of TV	10:00 p.m. Snack: Air-popped popcorn, chamomile tea
11:00 p.m. Collapse in bed, sleep fitfully	11:00 p.m. Snuggling with husband, sleep soundly

Fatigue-Busting Homework 101

I suggest two homework assignments to help kick-start your new energy program.

1 Keep a journal Chart your energy level on a scale of 1 to 10 for each hour of the day. Note how much and how well you slept the night before, how much you exercised, and what you ate, how much, and when. Then look for patterns. Knowing your highs and lows can help you work with your energy, maximizing your peak hours and nurturing yourself during the lows. For example, do you notice that your energy is good in the early morning, but sags midafternoon? If so, choose menial jobs, like unloading the dishwasher or folding clothes during slump times and use your high-energy hours for creative work (and lovemaking!!). Does your energy level vary depending on how much sleep, exercise or coffee you have that day? Use that information to design a plan for avoiding the energy drainers and emphasizing the energy boosters, based on the tips I'm about to tell you.

❷ **Buy a small notebook** Every morning take one minute to write down five reasons why you deserve to take good care of yourself today. This will help focus your attention on the positive and is a clear reminder of how important it is to nurture yourself so you have the energy to nurture others. Finally, keeping those reasons in a notebook makes it easy to look back on the thoughts you've had over the past year. It is a moment to be grateful, and that gratitude is a part of feeling positive, energized, appreciative and sexy.

QUICK FIX
energizers

Sometimes you just need a quick-fix energy jolt. Try these tricks to liven your day:

1. Take a brisk, 10-minute walk outside in the sunlight, which revs you up and is a natural aphrodisiac, as it reduces levels of sex-inhibiting hormones.

2. Sniff peppermint or jasmine. Both alter brain waves and help boost energy.

3. Turn on some upbeat music and dance. (Suggestions: Aretha Franklin's "Chain of Fools" or "Think," Rod Stewart's "Maggie May," Michael Jackson's "Beat It," Justin Timberlake's "Sexy Back," Guns N' Roses' "Welcome to the Jungle," Celine Dion's "I'm Alive" or Beyoncé's "Crazy in Love")

4. Laugh, really hard and for real.

5. Act as if. Stand up straight. Smile. Walk with confidence. Act as if you are feeling your oats and it's likely you'll feel more energized.

The Morning Routine

Terry was a breakfast skipper. "As soon as my feet hit the ground in the morning, I'm at a full run, so breakfast was an easy corner to cut. Besides, I wasn't even hungry, so why waste the calories?"

Big mistake. Spacing your meals, starting with breakfast, is one of the six S-Ex-Y Diet guidelines. The morning meal not only jump-starts your day, it jump-starts your mood, energy, mind and metabolism.

People who eat breakfast within the first two hours after getting up:

- have more energy
- have a more sustained good mood
- perform better at school and work
- sleep better at night, which means they wake up the next day more energized and happy
- learn faster
- are more creative
- pay closer attention
- are more focused throughout the day
- score better on memory tests

Breakfast lowers stress hormones to calm you through the morning hours. You will be less prone to uncontrollable food cravings and have a much easier time losing weight and, more importantly, maintaining the weight loss. In fact, 9 out of every 10 people who lose weight and keep it off eat breakfast almost every day. By contrast, breakfast skippers are four times as likely

> **Breakfast lowers stress hormones to calm you through the morning hours.**

to battle the bulge. It is also impossible to meet all your nutritional needs if you skip breakfast. With all those benefits, it is no surprise that people who eat breakfast also have more energy, desire and interest in sex. But I'm not talking doughnuts and coffee.

Barbara, a freelance writer in New Jersey, came face-to-face with how important breakfast was at the beginning of her career. "I was 23 years old, had just returned from a college job in Paris and was working for a major magazine in New York. I had been there a few weeks when my boss signaled me to come into her office. She said, 'It occurs to me that you are a little dumb in the morning. Are you eating breakfast?' It was a major turning point in my life. Up until then, I was totally unaware of my diet. My eating habits were awful. I skipped breakfast or grabbed a handful of cereal and a can of soda. And who else would think to eat a bag of thawed dinner rolls—uncooked?! I was young, but already was huffing and puffing up the stairs from the subway. That wake-up call got me eating breakfast. A little yogurt, fruit, an occasional egg. It changed my life. I started noticing a newfound energy, which motivated me to keep making more changes in how I ate. Now I'm not even tempted to eat greasy, bad food. I have so much energy, feel great, am never sick and am almost always in a great mood. I never had any of that before.

The Ménage à Trois Breakfast

What you do every day will have a far greater impact on your energy and sexiness than what you do once in a while. So, your goal for every morning is to restock your energy stores and set the stage for a day of boundless energy. The perfect breakfast is the Ménage à Trois breakfast (the Threesome breakfast). The three participants in this meal are:

1. A whole grain: to provide needed high-quality carbs for mental energy during the morning hours.

2. A little protein: to keep you satiated and maintain even blood sugar levels throughout the morning.

3. Two colorful fruits and/or vegetables: to provide a hefty dose of antioxidants, which protect delicate brain tissue from damage.

This breakfast is based on the authentic foods in the S-Ex-Y Diet and emphasizes the magic threesome for weight loss: fiber, protein and fluid, which fill you up before they fill you out. If you are overweight, dropping a few pounds by eating the Ménage à Trois breakfast is critical to upping your energy. People who are overweight are much more prone to fatigue and sleep problems than their lean friends, which makes sense. Imagine carrying a 20-, 30- or 100-pound bag of sand around all day. Now imagine how much more energy you would have if you put the bag down. As overweight people lose weight, their energy returns and their sleep improves. The Ménage à Trois breakfast with those three weight-loss ingredients is one giant step toward dropping that extra weight and keeping it off.

In spelling out the details of the Ménage à Trois breakfast to Terry, I told her to choose:

1 Whole Grains Carbs are especially important at this morning meal, since it has been 8 to 12 hours since you last ate. During that time, the body used much of its stored carbs just keeping you alive. Terry felt fine at first with a cup of coffee in her system and some sleep under her belt, but she was running on energy fumes and it affected her ability to think, work and say "no" to ice cream and chips later in the day. All grains supply the glucose your brain and body need to restock your fuel stores, but only whole grains keep blood sugar levels even throughout the morning, and supply lots of vitamins, minerals, fiber and phytonutrients not found in refined grains.

29

CEREAL *rules*

Don't be fooled by brands that say "Made with whole grain" or "A good source of whole grain." Even Cocoa Puffs is made with whole grains. Instead, flip the box over and check the Nutrition Facts panel. A rule of thumb is that the higher the sugar, the lower the fiber. Remember the number 5. You want cereals with: **no more than 5 grams of sugar** and **at least 5 grams of fiber**.

The less processed, the more filling a cereal will be and the longer it will "stick with you" through the morning. You want cereals made from 100% whole grains and ones that taste great, such as

1 Kashi Autumn Wheat

2 Barbara's Organic Grain Shop

3 Food for Life's Ezekial 4:9 Original

4 Nature's Path Organic Heritage Os

5 Shredded Wheat

2 Lean Protein Low-fat protein is low in the artery-clogging, energy-draining saturated fats found in greasier fare, such as whole milk, bacon and sausage. It also has staying power to keep you full and satisfied through the morning hours. (People who complain about being hungry all day when they eat breakfast typically have had an all-carb meal, such as a granola bar and fruit.) When choosing milk or soymilk as a source of protein, grab brands fortified with vitamin D and the omega-3 fat DHA, since these nutrients fight fatigue, help reduce pain and headaches, and boost mood. Other protein options include nuts or nut butters, eggs or egg substitutes, low-fat cheese, salmon, fat-free or low-fat cottage cheese and Canadian bacon. Plain, nonfat yogurt also is a great source of lean protein, and its probiotics (healthy bugs such as L-acidophilus or bifidus) promote energy in people battling fatigue.

3 Colorful Produce Antioxidants that protect your brain and tissues from damage are in the pigment or color of fruits and vegetables. The more color, the more antioxidants. Selections are endless and include berries, watermelon, tomatoes, spinach, apricots and juices such as carrot, orange and grapefruit.

Jump on the breakfast bandwagon. It will take about two to three weeks to reset your appetite clock and see an a boost in energy. But I guarantee you will feel better! Just ask Camille. "I've always been a breakfast eater. But what I once considered a healthy breakfast, like an omelet with buttered toast, I realized had too much fat. I inevitably was hungry and ate too much later in the day. Now I have fiber-rich oatmeal or another whole-grain cereal topped with a few almonds, fruit such as blackberries and skim milk. This breakfast is so filling and it keeps me going all morning long!"

Midmorning Quickie

Want to feel sexy all day long? The best way to keep energy flowing is to stop and refuel on a regular basis (S-Ex-Y Diet Guideline #3), something Terry frequently forgot to do. That means a midmorning snack about three to four hours after breakfast. Three minimeals and a few snacks throughout the day keep your appetite under control, rather than it controlling you. Eat when you are comfortably hungry and you'll choose the right fatigue-fighting foods. Wait until you are ravenous and you'll eat too much of all the wrong stuff. There is nothing in a vending machine that will fight fatigue, so carry Quickie snacks, based on a few rules:

1 **Mix quality carbs with protein** Carbs provide brain fuel, while protein fills you up and maintains blood sugar. Keep it low-fat and about 200 calories. Frisky Quickies include:

- A 6-ounce tub of low-fat yogurt and a piece of fruit.
- A small pouch of trail mix (Cheerios, nuts and dried fruit).
- String cheese with whole-grain crackers.
- A glass of DHA-fortified soymilk and grapes.
- Hummus with sliced red bell peppers and half a whole-grain pita.
- A sliced apple, 1 ounce Brie and 3 whole-grain crackers.
- Low-fat ricotta cheese with a chopped fig.

2 **Add a drink** Fatigue is the first sign of dehydration. By the time you're thirsty, you're already dehydrated. If it takes a glass of water to quench your thirst, then drink two or three glasses to rehydrate. The best bet is to front-load fluids by drinking a glass of water every hour throughout the day. Flavor it with a slice of lemon or a sprig of mint to make it more tempting to drink. Oh, and don't forget fruit as a source of fluids. Watermelon is 92% water; a large slice has the equivalent of a glass of water!

3 **De-sugar it** A sugary soft drink, candy bar or cookie might give you a quick surge of energy, but that burst turns to bust within an hour or two. One study found that a sweet snack perked people up in the short term but left them more tense an hour later, while a 10-minute brisk walk left them both energized and calmer for the next two hours.

To beat the bonk, steer clear of sugar. That doesn't mean you must give up sweets. Just focus on fruit instead of added sugar, such as cottage cheese with orange slices or a slice of turkey with cranberry chutney and fat-free cream cheese on whole-grain crackers.

A DOZEN MÉNAGE À TROIS breakfasts

1. A whole-grain freezer waffle, topped with lemon yogurt and fresh berries.

2. A toasted whole-grain English muffin, topped with smoked salmon, a scrambled egg and a thick slice of tomato. Serve with Tropicana orange juice.

3. Half a toasted whole-grain bagel, topped with peanut butter, sesame seeds and dried tart cherries. Serve with apple slices and a glass of DHA-fortified low-fat milk.

4. A slice of whole-grain crusty bread, topped with low-fat ricotta cheese and cherry tomatoes. Serve with grapefruit or carrot juice.

5. A bowl of whole-grain cereal, with vanilla yogurt, nuts and dried fruit. Serve with sliced cantaloupe.

6. Cook brown rice in DHA-fortified low-fat milk. Sprinkle with nuts, dried fruit and cinnamon. Serve with chopped mango and kiwi.

7. In a parfait glass, layer low-fat cottage cheese, pineapple, canned apricots and toasted wheat germ.

8. The Nibbler: 1 sliced apple, 1 ounce low-fat cheese, 1 ounce walnuts, olives and a slice of whole-wheat French bread.

9. Fill a whole-grain Mission Life Balance tortilla with almond butter, fresh berries and orange zest, and roll into a burrito. Serve with pomegranate juice.

10. Fill a whole-grain Mission Life Balance tortilla with scrambled egg substitute, low-fat cheese, black beans, corn and salsa. Serve with tomato juice.

11. Cook old-fashioned rolled oats or barley in low-fat milk. Toss in orange zest, dried cherries, cinnamon or nutmeg. Serve with orange slices. (Pack the cooked barley into a tight storage container and refrigerate. It will hold together so that you can slice it into "patties" and lightly fry those patties in nonstick cooking spray to make them crispy on the outside.)

12. Grab 'n' Go: A hard-boiled egg, whole-wheat French bread and an apple.

Midday Mojo Maintenance

On a typical day, Terry skipped breakfast, grabbed takeout for lunch, gulped down more coffee midafternoon, then attacked dinner like a ravenous wolf. With her hectic schedule, she'd forgotten the first and foremost rule—food is fuel. Just as you recharge your cell phone or laptop, you must regularly recharge your body's batteries or your main squeeze (that would be your body) sputters, spurts and conks out midday. Of course, if you skip breakfast, there is nothing you can eat midday that will bring back the energy you have lost. In that case, the best you can do is struggle through the day one way or the other, then tomorrow start the day right by eating a Ménage à Trois breakfast. Assuming you've started the morning right, then the goal by noon is to maintain your energy and avoid slumps midday.

The Twosome Lunch

Breakfast is all about business, but a S-Ex-Y Diet lunch can have a little thrill factor as long as you follow these two energizing rules:

1 **Keep it light** In keeping with S-Ex-Y Diet Guideline #5 (Remember that size matters), a heavy meal makes you sleepy and spacey. The heavier or fattier the meal, the bigger the slump. It's a delicate balancing act, where a little food gives you lots of energy, but eat too much and you crash. Consider *fat* a nickname for fatigue.

Terry's fatty fast-food lunch also set her up for an ice cream binge that night. A neurotransmitter called galanin rises around noontime and turns on cravings for fat. The more fat you eat, the more galanin you produce, which makes you want even more fat. Order Wendy's chicken caesar salad (8+ teaspoons of fat) or a chicken quesadilla at Taco Bell (7 teaspoons of fat), and galanin levels are jammed into high gear, increasing the likelihood that you'll finish off the Ho Hos tonight.

2 **Add a little protein** Don't focus solely on carbs. A high-carbohydrate lunch, no matter how healthy (such as pasta primavera and a spinach salad) raises brain levels of the nerve chemical serotonin, which leaves you relaxed and even sleepy. A nap with your sweetie on Saturday is great, but if you have a job interview or a project to complete during the week, the last thing you need is a tanked energy level.

A light 'n' low-fat Twosome lunch in line with S-Ex-Y Diet guidelines and guaranteed to keep you frisky would be:

- A turkey sandwich on whole-grain bread (try avocado, hummus, pesto, mustard or tapenade instead of mayo), a tossed salad (dressing on the side) and a piece of fruit.
- A whole-grain tortilla filled with leftover baked sweet potato chunks, low-fat cheese, black beans and bottled black bean and roasted corn salsa. Serve with baby carrots.
- A large tomato filled with tuna salad (use low-fat mayo), served with whole-grain bread sticks and a glass of DHA-fortified low-fat milk.
- A slice of Passionate Peppered Pizza (in the Recipe section). Serve with watermelon cubes.

Spice up lunch with herbs, such as rosemary, peppermint or basil, which contain a central nervous system stimulant called cineole. Fresh or dried, these herbs might give you a mild pick-me-up. Mix rosemary into your tuna salad, peppermint into your iced tea and basil on top of the pizza. (While bee pollen flunked the energy-boost test, there is some evidence that the herbs gotu kola and ginkgo biloba fight brain fatigue.)

Ironing Out Fatigue

Another cause of Terry's bone-numbing tiredness was iron deficiency. It didn't show up on the bloodwork because the doctor had checked only for anemia. You can be iron-deficient for months, years or even decades without being so deficient that it progresses to anemia, yet the symptoms are the same. You're tired, can't think straight, live on caffeine and might battle sleep issues. Iron is the key oxygen-carrier in the body. Low iron means you literally suffocate the tissues (and brain), which is the fast track to fatigue, poor concentration, reduced work performance and a squelched sex drive.

Women have almost twice the daily requirement for iron as men, but consume half as much food as men do. As a result, as many as 80% of exercising women and 20% of women in general are iron-deficient. Women who eat little or no red meat are at particular risk, because about 30% of the iron in meat (called heme iron) is absorbed, compared to only 2% to 7% of the nonheme iron in dried beans, whole grains, dark green vegetables and eggs. That means you must eat 4 to 15 times the servings of kidney beans (at ⅔ cup a serving) to match the iron absorbed from 3 ounces of red meat.

What can you do? First, get feisty. Active women should request more sensitive tests for tissue iron levels, including serum ferritin, transferrin saturation and total iron binding capacity (TIBC). A serum ferritin value below 20 mcg/L or a TIBC value greater than 360 mcg/dL signals iron deficiency. Women who exercise more than three hours a week, have been pregnant in the past two years, menstruate heavily or consume less than 2,500 calories daily are at particular risk. (It's unlikely you'll need a supplement if you are a man or postmenopausal woman, so check with a physician before adding extra iron to your supplement plan.)

If you are deficient, your physician will likely prescribe iron supplements. In addition, consume several servings daily of iron-rich foods. Iron intake also is a balance between iron promoters and iron inhibitors. So,

1 Combine a vitamin C–rich food with an iron-rich food, such as orange juice and a bean burrito. Vitamin C boosts iron absorption and counteracts some of the inhibitors in foods, such as phytates in whole grains.

2 Mix small amounts of heme iron in red meat with large amounts of nonheme to boost nonheme iron absorption. Extra-lean beef with chili beans, pork in a vegetable stir-fry and spaghetti with meatballs are examples.

3 Cook in a cast-iron skillet. The iron leaches out of the pot and into the food.

4 Select iron-fortified foods.

5 Drink tea and coffee between meals, since compounds called tannins in these beverages block iron absorption. Allow 90 minutes between a cup of coffee or tea and a meal to avoid the "tannin effect."

6 Take iron supplements on an empty stomach to improve absorption. If it causes stomach upset, try taking the supplement in small, divided doses.

Evening Energizers

Your goal from lunchtime to bedtime is to maximize evening relaxation and night-time sleep. Living with a sleep deficit will undermine your best efforts to eat right and feel energized, alert and sexy. Even shortchanging sleep by an hour and a half is enough to lose up to a third of your normal alertness the next day. Lack of sleep leads to depression, stress, anxiety, fatigue, poor concentration and memory, weight gain, high blood pressure, elevated stress hormones and possibly even breast cancer and stroke. It more than doubles the risk for diabetes and increases heart disease risk by 40%. Lab tests show changes in hormones and nerve function in sleep-deprived 30-year-olds

> 66 *You might think you are too busy to get enough sleep, but really you are too busy not to.* 99

that mimic those of people in their 70s. In other words, lack of enough sleep increases your chances of facing The Big Sleep at an earlier age. Being sleep-deficient lowers levels of human growth hormone, which leads to muscle loss, suppressed immunity and increased body fat. It also might cause a drop in testosterone, which further lowers your sex drive and makes you crabby, moody and disinterested in socializing, which means no dates for you!

If you need an alarm clock to wake up, you fall asleep within five minutes of hitting the pillow, you get drowsy listening to lectures or at meetings or you feel tired or listless during the week, then you are sleep-deprived. Chuck the excuses. You might think you are too busy to get enough sleep, but really you are too busy not to.

Are You Short on Sleep?

How do you know if you are sleep deprived? Respond to the following statements with a yes or no. Three or more yeses means you are one of the many sleep walkers who have become so used to grogginess they don't even know they are tired!

If it wasn't for the alarm clock, I'd sleep past my wake up time.

It is a major effort to get out of bed in the morning.

I have been known to hit the snooze button more than once on weekdays.

I often feel tired and cranky during the week.

I find myself not listening, having trouble concentrating or forgetting important things.

I often fall asleep for more than an hour as a passenger in a car.

I often nod off in boring meetings or lectures.

Plunk me in a chair in front of television and I am asleep in no time.

Many times I'm asleep within five minutes of turning off the light.

I am often drowsy when driving or doing routine chores.

I often sleep extra hours on weekends, if given the chance.

Caffeine Caresses

Most people know that caffeine is a minishot of speed. Within minutes of entering the bloodstream, caffeine amps up the nervous system, helping you think faster, remember more, feel energized and even be happier. A study from the University of Michigan in Ann Arbor found that women who drank a cup of coffee every day reported having more sex than nondrinkers, maybe because caffeine stimulates the nervous system and boosts blood flow, making them more sensitive to touch and quick to respond.

On the other hand, caffeine doesn't really supply energy—it robs your body of it, because it revs your engine without giving it fuel. In no time, the false energy is replaced with real fatigue. You go back for another cup of coffee (or Red Bull, cola or tea) and wind up riding a roller coaster of highs and lows. In addition, compounds in teas and coffee (caffeinated, decaffeinated, herbal, black, green, red or white teas) block iron absorption by up to 90%. Worse yet, combine sweets with coffee, as Terry did with her midday snack of coffee and a muffin, and you have a double whammy guaranteed to leave you running on fumes.

Don't get me wrong. You can have coffee or tea or any caffeinated beverage or food, just put a lid on the amount. A cup or two in the morning is fine. But fueling your day with coffee is like having one foot on the accelerator and one foot on the brake: Sooner or later you will strip the gears. Also, caffeine lingers in the system for hours. That monster drink you had at 4 p.m. could be the reason you toss and turn at midnight. Even a coffee-flavored yogurt can have the caffeine equivalent of a half cup of coffee.

The solution? Keep your coffee consumption to a few cups before 2 p.m. Or drink a small amount (like 2 ounces) of a caffeinated beverage several times a day, rather than all at once. Then cut off the caffeine by late afternoon. That will give you a gentler energy boost, but is less likely to disrupt sleep.

The Evening Meal

If you want to maintain your mojo until bedtime and then sleep like a baby, you must eat right at night. That's what Rupa found. "I typically eat really healthy and have lots of energy. But every so often I'll have the week from hell. Late-night dinners with plates piled with heavy, salty foods, mixed with lots of wine and fats from dessert. The next day I typically have to leave the office early because I am so tired! I literally crash and feel sick. High stress, late meals and heavy foods are the absolute worst mix for me!"

> **66** *A high-fat meal lowers testosterone by up to 50%.* **99**

Big dinners make you temporarily drowsy, but they also prolong digestive action, which keeps you awake. A high-fat meal lowers testosterone by up to 50%, which can really put a squelch on lovemaking that night! Instead, try eating your biggest meals before midafternoon and eat a light evening meal. Include some chicken, fish or extra-lean meat at dinner to help curb middle-of-the-night snack attacks.

Spicy or gas-forming foods can aggravate sleep problems. Dishes seasoned with garlic, chilies, cayenne or other hot spices can cause nagging heartburn or indigestion, while the flavor-enhancer MSG (monosodium glutamate) causes vivid dreaming and restless sleep in some people. Gas-forming foods, such as cucumbers or beans, as well as eating too fast, cause abdominal discomfort, which in turn interferes with sound sleep. In short: Avoid spicy foods at dinnertime. Limit your intake of gas-forming foods to the morning hours and thoroughly chew food to avoid gulping air. Also, steer clear of fatty red meats and sauces that make you sluggish, as well as salty foods that dehydrate you.

Items that help bring on the zzzz's include:

- **Real food** Whole grains, dark green leafies, legumes and nuts in the S-Ex-Y Diet are high in magnesium, a mineral that plays a key role in regulating sleep, and that might help stop restless leg syndrome.

- **Fatty fish** The omega-3 fats in fish, including EPA and DHA, boost both physical and mental energy, and possibly even improve sleep. That's why "Get wet and wild twice a week" is one of the six tenets of the S-Ex-Y Diet. Complement a salmon steak with a baked sweet potato and a tossed salad for the perfect evening meal.

- **Lean protein** Skinless chicken breast, seafood or nonfat milk products are rich in vitamin B_{12}, which helps regulate melatonin, the body's sleep hormone.

- **Lavender** The scent eases anxiety, headaches and fatigue, and prepares you for a restful sleep. It also increases slow-wave sleep, the very deep sleep where heart rate slows and muscles relax. Along with sprinkling lavender water on your sheets or tucking petals under your pillow, try infusing lavender into sauces for poached pears or ice cream.

- **Melatonin-rich foods** Tart dried cherries, bananas, brown rice and sweet corn contain small amounts of this sleep-enhancing hormone.

The Nightcap

Alcohol is a false friend. A nightcap might help you *go* to sleep, but not *stay* asleep. You'll sleep less soundly and wake up more tired as a result. Alcohol and other depressants suppress a phase of sleep called REM (Rapid Eye Movement), where most dreaming occurs. It is in REM sleep where 70% of women and nearly all men have their lively sex dreams! Less REM sleep is associated with more night awakenings and restless sleep. A glass or two of wine with dinner is fine, but avoid drinking any alcohol within two hours of bedtime and *never* mix alcohol with sleeping pills!

Bedtime Story

The evening snack might be the best alternative to sleeping pills. A high-carbohydrate snack (remember the G-Spot snack from Chapter 1?), such as whole-grain crackers and fruit, air-popped popcorn or whole-wheat toast and jam triggers the release of the brain chemical serotonin, which aids sleep. A light carbohydrate-rich snack that supplies no more than 30 grams of carbohydrate before bedtime helps some people sleep longer and more soundly. *(See Chapter 1, page 17, for more all-carb snack ideas.)*

Ginseng: Might help regulate the sleep-wake cycle, and some herbalists swear that ginseng has aphrodisiac properties, but it also causes nervousness in some people and has hormonelike effects, so consult a physician before use. Siberian ginseng might be safer than Asian ginseng. Dose: 1–2 grams of the root or 200–600 milligrams of extract.

Valerian: Might have a tranquilizing effect, relaxing muscles and suppressing the nervous system. Few side effects. Dose: 400–900 milligrams.

Kava kava: Might have a sedative and relaxing effect, but should not be taken with antidepressants or with alcohol. Dose: 180–210 milligrams.

Melatonin: A hormonelike substance produced in a brain center called the pineal gland that helps regulate sleep. Supplements might improve light sleep, but may not induce a deep, restful sleep. Dose: 1–3 milligrams.

GABA and 5-HTP: This combo might help you fall asleep faster and sleep longer. No firm recommendations have been set, but some studies have used 2 grams/day of GABA and 100 milligrams of 5-HTP.

What about a glass of warm milk? Milk is a good source of the building block for serotonin, an amino acid called tryptophan. However, the protein in milk blocks tryptophan entry into the brain. No serotonin is made when you drink milk. However, any warm beverage, like a warm cup of milk or a cup of chamomile tea, does soothe and relax, and provides a feeling of satiety, which might help facilitate sleep. Add a bit of vanilla extract to milk to evoke a feeling of security or comfort.

Nighty Night

Finish off this energizing day with a sleep-lover's routine by turning a Grand Central bedroom, filled with lounging pets, blaring TVs and left-over paperwork into a peaceful sanctuary. Beds are for cuddling, intimate talks, lovemaking and sleep. Hit the sack at about the same time every night (and get up at the same time in the morning). Experts swear that this routine helps set the body's sleep-wake cycle. Take a warm shower or bubble bath, slip into something comfy and between clean sheets, turn off the lights and finish the day with sex, which raises endorphins that have a soporific effect.

In addition, a major difference between good sleepers and poor sleepers is not what they do at bedtime, but what they did all day. Good sleepers exercise and use every opportunity to move. Physical activity helps a person cope with daily stress and tires the body so it is ready for sleep at night. (*See Chapter 9.*)

Terry slowly changed her diet and daily routine and now has all the energy she needs to enjoy her life, work, kids and hubby. "I used to look at my husband like he was crazy when he'd get amorous. I was so tired I couldn't remember my name some days, let alone feel like a roust in the hay. But now I'm the one taking his hand and leading him to the bedroom. You'd better believe I made a follow-up appointment with my doctor and let him know my energy had nothing to do with my age—it was all about how I was taking care of myself!"

Slump-Proof Your Life

There is no excuse to put up with fatigue as a lifestyle. Take care of yourself by eating the S-Ex-Y Diet, having a Ménage à Trois breakfast, a Twosome lunch, lots of water and a few super-nutritious Quickie snacks throughout the day, then keep your evening meal light, make sure to include some vigorous activity during the day and have a G-Spot snack just before bed. I promise you'll be one sexy lover 24/7 in no time!

3

DO YOU THINK
you're sexy?

THE PROMISE

Within **THREE WEEKS** of making these changes, you will

✓ Notice improvements in your memory, reaction times and thinking ability.

✓ Notice positive changes in your mood and emotions.

✓ Cope better with stress.

✓ Show lower inflammation in the body, reducing your risk for all age-related diseases.

In **SIX MONTHS**, you will

✓ Notice continued improvements in memory and sexual function.

✓ Feel more hopeful and experience more even, positive moods throughout the day.

✓ Drop a few pounds and inches around your waistline.

In **ONE YEAR**, you will

✓ Remember where you put your keys, the dog's name and the title of that movie.

✓ Feel more yourself, happier and calmer or less agitated.

✓ Be able to cope better than you did a year ago.

✓ Have dropped a few more pounds.

In **THIRTY YEARS**, you will

✓ Think more clearly and remember more than your friends.

✓ Still be enjoying a romp in the hay with your sweetie.

I was on a panel of experts in New York about to report on the latest research on how diet can improve mind, mood and memory. The moderator had just stood up to announce the start of the event. The audience of reporters, editors and other media people were finishing their lunches and eager to hear the latest research on how diet, exercise and lifestyle improve mind and memory.

I leaned over to my colleague on the panel, an expert on brain research, and quietly asked his opinion on what he felt was the most important habit we should cultivate—besides exercise and increasing our intake of antioxidants and the omega-3s—to protect our minds and stay mentally sharp throughout life. I expected a somber answer, such as "Drink red, not white, wine" or "Take an extra dose of ginkgo." Instead, this brilliant, soft-spoken man looked me right in the eye, and with a sincere and honest expression on his face whispered, "Sex."

Not only did his response take me by surprise, giving me the best laugh of the day, but it also got me thinking. Regular great rousts in the hay with someone dear to your heart is one of the most important habits for keeping you mentally young. OK. I get that. But to turn on the lust in the first place requires a brain fine-tuned and ready for action. If your brain isn't in the mood, the rest of you won't be, either. It's a chicken-and-egg scenario—thinking sexy generates more opportunity for sex, which generates a younger, more eager brain, which means...wooo hoo, more sex.

Luckily, you have much more control over your memory and mind than you probably imagine, which means following the advice below can only be a plus for your sex life.

Your #1 Sex Organ

The first few times you forget where you put your keys, can't remember a word midsentence, or the name of that actor—"Oh, what's his name, he was in that movie...oh, you remember, that movie with the big whatchamacallit, you know, that big fish with a fin on its back"—you might not think much of it. Maybe it's just a bad day or you didn't get enough sleep last night or you are distracted by work, the kids, the phone. Over time, you start to notice a pattern. You find yourself walking around the house looking for something, but now can't remember what it is. Then your daughter tells you those glasses you are searching for are

> **66** *Everything you know about brain aging is probably wrong.* **99**

on your head. You start thinking, "Didn't I used to be smarter than this?" From there, it's easy to think you're on the one-way highway to Forgetville.

First off, your memory was never perfect, so get over it. Every one of us has senior moments, even if we aren't seniors. Second, your memory lapses are probably just a result of mental overload. Multitasking can overload that complex computer in your head. Even if there is some loss of clarity, it doesn't mean you're in the early stages of dementia or that it will progress. In fact, everything you know about brain aging is probably wrong.

As Good As It Gets

Your brain is not destined to get fuzzy. Even if there is a history of dementia in your family, that has very little to do with you. Genetics are only part of the equation: 66% of how smart you are and will be in the future has to do with how you choose to take care of yourself yesterday, today and tomorrow. The belief that brain cells can't regenerate, that there is a finite number, which wither, dwindle and die over time—leading to memory loss, dementia and even Alzheimer's—is outdated and just plain wrong.

Scientists now recognize that the brain is amazingly resilient and "plastic," which means it has the ability to tweak its structure and function. Throughout life, the brain continues to form new cells (called neurons) and activate alternative pathways to compensate for aging or damaged parts. Memory loss is *not* a decree. The one in three people who battle even minor memory loss typically can blame that mental fog more on lifestyle and other health issues, such as high blood pressure, heart disease or diabetes, than on genes. Even the 15% who suffer senile dementia might have slowed, stopped or even reversed the disease with a change in diet and lifestyle.

> 66 *Your brain is only as good as what you feed it.* 99

Your brain is only as good as what you feed it. Make stupid lifestyle choices, such as eating a high-saturated-fat diet, sitting like a lump on the couch, smoking or refusing to learn new things as you age, and you are asking for a dramatic decline in brain-cell numbers and their connections, which means fewer cells to store memory and fewer connections between cells to retrieve them. That increases your chances for dementia and Alzheimer's 16-fold.

Or get smart and follow the S-Ex-Y Diet guidelines, exercise daily and adopt a few memory-boosting habits, and you literally increase the size of your brain, the number of neurons and the number of connections between nerve cells. That translates into an astonishing improvement in mind, memory and mood both today and down the road, which gives you more years of feeling sexy and ready for action! And probably more creative in the bedroom, too. In short, the problem is not so much that the mind fails, but that we fail to keep our minds engaged and nourished. *(Take the "How Sexy Is Your Mind?" quiz on page 194 to see how well you are caring for your brain.)*

Brainiac 101

Your brain is an absolutely, no-doubt-about-it, miraculous organ. Weighing in at about 3 pounds and about the size of a small cantaloupe, it contains 100 billion cells, with each of those neurons sprouting up to 100,000 connections or links (called synapses) to other neurons. Pluck out a tiny piece of the brain as little as a grain of rice and you are holding 1 million neurons, 10 billion synapses and 20 miles of nerve tissues!

The entire brain lights up for sex, including centers for all five senses—visual, hearing, smell, taste and touch. Housed in the center of the brain, the limbic system is a particularly important area to nourish. This is where body meets mind and where thoughts meet emotions. Here you will find:

1 **The hippocampus** This is the memory and learning center and the first to go when a person develops Alzheimer's. Bigger means better when it comes to memory. The right diet, exercise and lifestyle increase the number of neurons in the hippocampus, pumping up its size, well into our 70s, while out-of-control stress, poor diet and being sedentary shrink this memory center.

2 **The amygdala** Here is where meaning is assigned to emotions, such as the warm and fuzzy memory of your first kiss or the appeal of those sexy thoughts a man has every 52 seconds. (There are 10 times as many nerves going north from this emotion center to the conscious, rational brain center—the cortex—than there are nerves going south, which explains why it is difficult to think rationally when it comes to love!)

3 **The hypothalamus** This is the switchboard that regulates how you respond to situations (like whether or not that come-on line at the bar resulted in a "Hello, Big Boy" or a "Get Lost, Loser"). Along with the hippocampus, the hypothalamus "lights up" during a woman's orgasm. Finally, it is a major control center for appetite, releasing most of the appetite-control chemicals, including serotonin, NPY and galanin.

4 **The pituitary** This is the master gland that sits next to the hypothalamus and tells other glands what to do, such as release testosterone as well as the hormones that regulate fertility, which in turn revs up your sexy center. It is no coincidence that the neurons that regulate sexuality and those that control eating are located next door to each other in the pituitary and hypothalamus.

5 **The insula** As the messenger between the limbic system and higher brain centers, the insula relays emotional information and sparks your cravings for sex. The more active this part of the limbic system, the more orgasms a woman is likely to have. Hmm.

All these compartments of the limbic system record, reorganize, synthesize and retrieve information, but only as well as they are fed and nurtured. It doesn't take a rocket scientist to figure out how important S-Ex-Y Diet Guideline #2 is: Feed your #1 sex organ—your brain!

As You Eat, So Shall You Think

In the short term, any and all diet advice to jump-start energy will also prevent mental fatigue. Eat the Ménage à Trois breakfast, drink ample water, have a Twosome lunch, a light and low-fat dinner, regularly supply your brain with its favorite fuel—glucose—drink a little but not too much caffeine and get enough iron if you are a woman, and I guarantee that your mind will do what it does best— think—throughout the day.

That's what Camille found when she took my advice to make a few changes in her diet. "I am eating lots more real food and a lot less junk these days. Who knew vegetables could make a girl so smart! I am much sharper than I used to be. I multitask much more efficiently. In fact, if you compare my mental acuity to picture quality, the image is sharper, more vivid, with deeper colors than when I ate less healthy."

You also can save and even improve brainpower in the long term. Your brain is a nutrient-needy organ, entirely made up of what you choose to feed it. Diet is the only place the brain gets the building blocks to run its highly sophisticated computer system, which in turn runs the whole body. Following the guidelines of the S-Ex-Y Diet will reduce inflammation, improve blood flow, protect against aging and disease, provide all the necessary building blocks for making and rejuvenating healthy brain cells throughout life, enhance brain-cell communication and maximize energy use. Trust me: Don't take your diet lightly—even one fatty meal has a subtle influence on your brain for up to 180 days! A grease-bomb burger also lowers testosterone levels in men, leaving them more interested in the recliner than the bedroom.

> 66 ... even one fatty meal has a subtle influence on your brain for up to 180 days! 99

It goes even further than that. If you don't follow the S-Ex-Y Diet guidelines (and exercise program outlined later), you can expect about a 5% decline in memory every decade after your 20s. A study from Case Western Reserve University in Cleveland found that people who did not take care of their minds in their 20s through 50s were three times more likely to develop Alzheimer's in their 60s and 70s. By contrast, seniors who eat right, move more and live well react and problem-solve just as quickly as people who are decades younger. If you don't want to be walking down Memory Lame in the future, you'd better start taking care of your brain now.

There's Nothing Sexy About Inflammation

Have you ever been so mad you could scream? Or punch a wall? Your heart races, your face turns red, your teeth clench. You feel as though you're on fire. Now think of your body's tissues and brain cells. They get enraged, too. But for different reasons. You don't feel those enraged tissues, but all the disease of aging, from heart disease and dementia to sexual problems like erectile dysfunction, have one underlying factor in common—inflammation. The good news is that you can slow, stop and possibly even reverse damage caused by inflammation by following the S-Ex-Y Diet, exercising and being a bit fussier about how you live.

The Inflamed Brain

The term *inflammation* comes from a Latin word meaning to "set a fire." It is the body's natural response to healing. Not to be confused with infection, inflammation is how the body contains infection and injury, while promoting repair of damaged tissue. You know inflammation by its outward signs: redness or flulike symptoms, such as fever or chills.

What's going on? Any damage to a tissue tells the immune system to send white blood cells to the area in an attempt to remove damaged cells, bacteria, toxins or irritants. These blood cells release hormonelike chemicals, called eicosanoids, that increase blood flow to the area, causing redness and warmth. They also cause leakage of fluid into the tissues, which is why a stubbed toe swells.

There are two types of inflammation: One is good and the other isn't. Acute inflammation works great for healing a cut finger or a bumped head. The white blood cells and their chemicals get in, do their job and get out.

But too much of a good thing leads to problems. Chronic inflammation damages, rather than repairs, tissues. When inflammation is too intense or prolonged, it produces diseases instead of healing. Tissues damaged by the wrong diet or lifestyle choice set up a constant irritant in the body, resulting in chronic inflammation that works silently under the surface, damaging arteries and tissues, leading to heart disease, dementia and even loss of libido.

Feed Your Head

Diet is a major player in whether or not you fight fire or fuel the flames. The eicosanoids released to fight infection come in two varieties—promoters and inhibitors. In a healthy body, those two forces are in balance, so inflammation occurs only when and where it is needed and stops when damage is repaired. But a system out of balance with too many damaging compounds constantly irritates tissues, leading to disease.

Your brain's promoting and inhibiting chemicals are made from fats in the diet. The fats consumed in safflower or corn oil are called omega-6 fats and they promote inflammation. A specific omega-6 fat, called arachidonic acid, found in meats, is a particularly potent promoter.

Other foods promote inflammation because they are irritants to the body's tissues, which then trigger the immune response. These brain-damaging foods include saturated fats in meat and fatty dairy products; refined grains and sugar; trans fats in processed and fast foods, potatoes and fried foods; palm or coconut oils; pastries; and processed meats like hot dogs (the nitrite additives in these luncheon meats are especially damaging).

Foods that put out the fire of inflammation are the foundation of the S-Ex-Y Diet. They include the omega-3 fats in fish oils and flaxseed, as well as extra-virgin olive oil, colorful fruits and vegetables, mushrooms, nuts, soy, whole grains, tea and certain spices, such as turmeric and ginger. Eat real, unprocessed foods most of the time and focus on plants and fatty fish and you will soothe the fires and stay brain-strong.

That's just what Brenda found out. We met on the Dr. Oz show. She needed to lose weight and I offered to help. Over the next few months, Brenda found that making a few simple changes in how she ate not only resulted in major weight loss, it also seriously improved her thinking. "Since our lifestyle changes, I have noticed a big difference in my memory. Before, I had to make notes in my phone, write calendar reminders and set alarms to remind me about important things. I don't need to do that anymore. I can keep my life organized in my head and find I remember just fine these days!"

GET-SMART
quickies

For a quick pick-me-up snack that fuels your brain and reduces inflammation, try:

- ⅓ cup mixed almonds, dried blueberries and Cheerios.
- Celery topped with tuna mixed with fat-free, plain yogurt with fresh herbs.
- Sliced apple with almond butter and a glass of low-sodium V8.
- A brown rice cake spread with pesto, topped with mackerel or sardines and diced tomatoes.
- 100% whole-grain crackers, topped with fat-free cream cheese, smoked salmon, cucumber slices and fresh dill.
- Chopped walnuts mixed into fat-free cream cheese and spread on dried apricot halves.
- Thick slices of banana topped with peanut butter and sprinkled with dried tart cherries and coconut.
- Orange and apple slices sprinkled with cinnamon. Serve with a 6-ounce tub of plain, nonfat yogurt.
- Thin-sliced whole-grain nut bread, topped with peanut butter and sliced strawberries.
- Red grapes, sliced almonds and craisins mixed into nonfat, Greek yogurt.
- Baby carrots, pea pods, red bell pepper slices and lightly steamed broccoli florets dunked in hummus.

The Fats of Life

Fats either plug or promote thinking, depending on which ones you choose. Besides escalating inflammation, saturated and trans fats pack on the pounds (we'll get to your waistline in Chapter 4) and clog arteries, including the ones to your brain. That seriously impairs oxygen flow to the brain, which is a bummer for memory and attention. End result: You are a dumb fathead! Combine saturated fat with sugar and you have a surefire way to suppress the hippocampus, which means you struggle with new information and learning doesn't come easily. And don't forget cholesterol. Too much cholesterol increases your chances of memory loss by up to 75%!

Don't get me wrong. Fat can be your best friend, if you make the right choices. You absolutely must keep your brain cells flexible and fluid if you want to be thinking sexy thoughts and acting on them with your lover for the rest of your life.

The Smart Fat

Your brain is very greasy, but in a good way. More than 60% of it is fat. Unlike the lazy fat stored on the hips or belly, fat in the brain is a worker bee. It makes up the cell membranes that surround each cell and the insulation sheath around neurons that allows thoughts to travel fast from one cell to another. The more fluid and flexible those membranes, the faster you react, the more you remember and the more creative and clever you are. All of which are great assets in the dating game! The right fats also produce anti-inflammatory eicosanoids that protect brain tissue from aging and boost serotonin levels, the feel-good brain chemical that soothes both mood and food cravings.

That's why the brain loves omega-3 fats, especially DHA. Omega-3 fats are the most fluid of all fats. Your body can't make them, so it is entirely dependent on your choosing the grilled salmon instead of the cheeseburger for lunch. Follow S-Ex-Y Diet Guideline #4 (Get wet and wild at least twice a week) by eating salmon, and the brain will greedily suck up and deposit DHA into its neurons. Nerve connections alone increase by almost a third by adding more DHA to the diet! The more DHA consumed, the more DHA is incorporated into brain tissue, and the smarter, more clever and creative you become and stay. Also, your brain will be less prone to gooey plaque that builds up around nerve cells leading to Alzheimer's. *(See Chapter 1.)*

This might explain why a DHA-rich diet lowers dementia risk by up to 60%. There is even preliminary evidence that DHA might help soothe and heal a brain that has suffered a trauma, such as in a car accident or on the football field. Oh, and did I mention that people are less angry, hostile or anxious, they sleep better, are less prone to outbursts of temper and have an easier time focusing when their brains are loaded with DHA? All of that most definitely will improve a person's love life!

You get the biggest bang for your buck with DHA, and maybe a bit of help from EPA. You'll get the least results from the omega-3 fat alpha linolenic acid, or ALA, in flax, walnuts, soy and other plants, which is great for the heart and circulation, and will help lower inflammation, but does nothing for boosting memory or lowering dementia risk. There is up to 30 times more DHA than EPA in tissues, and up to 97% of the omega-3s in the brain are DHA. Also, DHA can be converted to EPA in the body, so you get two for the price of one with that fat.

How much do you need? As S-Ex-Y Diet Guideline #4 says, aim for two servings of fatty fish a week, such as salmon, mackerel, herring or sardines, and choose foods fortified with an algal-based, contaminant-free DHA. It will say *life'sDHA* on the label. If you supplement, choose one that contains at least 1 gram of a combination of DHA and EPA, or one that supplies at least 220 milligrams of DHA.

That's just a minimum. The Memory Improvement with Docosahexaenoic Acid Study found that 900 milligrams of DHA significantly boosted memory and mental function within six months, which suggests that, in the case of DHA, more might be better. Make sure to keep it coming, since studies on animals show that DHA levels take a nosedive within three months of low intake.

Antioxidants are Brain Candy

Want to seriously improve your mind and sexy self? Then combine DHA with S-Ex-Y Diet Guideline #1: Have an antioxidant orgy. That means platefuls of colorful fruits and vegetables, starting with at least 9 servings a day. The DHA will build a better brain and the antioxidants will protect it from damage.

The culprit here is oxygen. While oxygen is the most important nutrient for life, it also has a dark side. Oxygen fragments, called oxidants or free radicals, are part of the air we breathe. They also are in fried foods, air pollution, tobacco smoke and sunlight, and are generated in the body during normal metabolism.

These oxidants are like street gangs attacking unsuspecting cells, cell membranes and even the genetic code within cells. Left unchecked, each cell in our body is attacked about 1,000 times a day. As cells are damaged or killed, the accumulating

WHERE DO YOU *find DHA?*
8th Continent Soymilk Complete
Apple bran muffins at Starbucks
Cabot 50% Reduced Fat Cheddar Cheese with omega-3 DHA
Crisco Puritan canola oil
Darigold SuperMilk 1% low-fat milk
Dr. Dave's Mega-O Vegetarian Truffles
Francesco Rinaldi ToBe Healthy sauces
Fujisan fresh sushi
Gold Circle Farm eggs
Horizon Little Blends yogurt
Horizon Milk with DHA Omega-3 (fat free, 2% and whole milk)
Horizon Lowfat Chocolate Milk plus DHA Omega-3
Minute Maid Enhanced Pomegranate Blueberry juice
Mission Life Balance Plus! tortillas (available in flour and whole wheat)
Pompeian OlivExtra Plus
Silk DHA Omega-3 & Calcium
Silk Plus DHA Omega-3 Fortified Soy Beverage
So Good Omega DHA milk (original and vanilla)

debris clogs tissues, while organs begin to break down. Oxidative damage is a major underlying cause of all age-related diseases, from cancer to dementia and Alzheimer's. It also initiates inflammation and reduces the ability to become sexually aroused.

The brain is particularly vulnerable to oxidative damage. It accounts for only 2% of ideal body weight, but consumes between 20% and 25% of the oxygen we inhale. Consequently, it generates more oxidants per gram of tissue than any other organ in the body. For example, the nerve chemicals that regulate appetite, such as serotonin and galanin discussed in Chapter 1, release massive amounts of oxidants every time they are released. The fluid and flexible fats in brain cell membranes are particularly vulnerable to oxidative attack. The onslaught over the course of years slowly kills brain cells, tangles their connections, causes a buildup of gooey plaque, damages blood vessels needed to feed neurons and shuts down brain activity. The more oxidants, the more damage and the greater your risk for thinking less like a steel trap and more like a sieve.

Fortunately, the body has an antioxidant or anti–free radical system to halt, or at least slow, oxidative damage. That system includes enzymes that act like a police force released into the cellular neighborhood to round up the oxidant street gangs. It also includes dietary antioxidant nutrients, such as vitamins E and C, beta-carotene, selenium and manganese, plus the phytonutrients (anthocyanins, polyphenols, carotenoids, flavonoids, etc.) in colorful fruits, vegetables, whole grains, nuts, seeds, legumes, red wine, herbs, cocoa powder and tea. The brain is smart enough to know that it needs a ton of protection, and will automatically concentrate these antioxidants if you eat them. For example, vitamin C is concentrated 15 times greater in the brain than in most other tissues if you eat lots of citrus and other C-rich foods.

The stronger your antioxidant arsenal, the more of these protective compounds are absorbed by the brain, the greater the brain protection and the more youthful your mind today and down the road. Learning, coordination, balance and attitude also improve. Antioxidants even reverse brain aging in some people. People who eat the most antioxidant-rich foods also have the best memories, the sharpest minds and the most creative ideas. Antioxidants aren't stored in the body. They must be constantly replenished by including at least 9 servings in the daily diet.

Antioxidant supplements help, but they aren't a shortcut to brain protection. Vitamin E supplements help prevent the gooey buildup around neurons associated with Alzheimer's, vitamin C pills improve memory and an extra dose of beta-carotene might help brain cells communicate. But the greatest brain protection comes from a mix of antioxidants that you get only from a wide variety of colorful, authentic (i.e., unprocessed) foods, which supply the right amounts and balance of the almost 1 million phytonutrients. Skip the lutein supplement or pills that tout a full serving of vegetables in every dose. That's hype, not help.

Stress: The Brain Drain

Stress is one of the biggest causes of memory loss. I'm not talking about fun stress, like learning to tango or speak Italian. It is chronic stress from worry, fretting, anxiety about money woes, self-esteem issues, time pressure, anger, loneliness, relationship problems and more. Bad stress releases chemicals and oxidants in such force that it can bring any brain to its knees. Blood pressure rises, immune function plummets, minute tears in the brain don't heal and inflammation has a free-for-all.

Stress causes the adrenal glands to release cortisol. High levels of this hormone cause inflammation, kill neurons, suppress or halt the formation of new brain cells and damage the hippocampus, the part of the brain critical to memory and learning. In fact, chronic stress can shrink the hippocampus by up to 14%! Stress also raises a compound in the blood, called homocysteine, that irritates blood vessels, setting up inflammation associated with dementia and sexual dysfunction. It triggers the release of another chemical, called norepinephrine, that puts a damper on libido. Waste products, including a compound called lipofusin, accumulate, blocking electrical activity in the brain and leading to cell death. Finally, stress increases the requirement for several nutrients, such as vitamin C, and drains the body of magnesium, a mineral that otherwise helps you cope with stress. As a result, the nutrient losses escalate the stress response and brain damage.

If you've ever been stressed out, you have suffered the immediate effects of this damage—poor concentration, muddled thinking and poor decision-making skills. You are distracted, spacey, forgetful. You repeatedly use the words "thingamajig" and "whatchamacallit." Needless to say, thoughts of sex fly out the window as cortisol levels rise. It is tough to think about being sexy or even being intimate when you are barely holding it all together. Sex feels like just one more thing that has to get done.

Maxed-Out Waistline

To make matters worse, when the going gets tough, the tough get hungry. Cortisol has a domino effect on most appetite-control chemicals in the brain, from serotonin to NPY, which stimulates cravings for sweet and greasy foods, like ice cream, pizza, sausage, hamburgers and chocolate. These foods soothe us and help calm us down, but the cortisol forces those incoming calories to be stored as fat around the middle. Even if you are typically a lean machine, chronic stress will increase ab flab. That spare tire in your 40s will triple your chances of having dementia later in life. In fact, according to a study from Northwestern University's Feinberg School of Medicine in Chicago, memory decreases for every one point increase in a middle-aged woman's body mass index (BMI), a measurement of body fat. The bottom line is that the brains of overweight people appear 16 years older and are considerably smaller than the brains of lean, fit people.

Stress-Busting S-Ex-Y Diet Tricks

Your brain is far too important to beat it up with stress. Do whatever it takes to calm down. Do it now! Meditate, get more sleep, do yoga, have a massage, get organized, declutter your life, put on upbeat music, breathe deeply, visualize peace, delegate, just say "no" to more work, use biofeedback, walk in the outdoors, garden, tell funny stories, get and give a foot rub or giggle daily. Best yet—a good lovemaking session is great for stress reduction, since orgasms, coupled with intimacy and physical closeness, drop cortisol levels like a skydiver without a parachute.

The S-Ex-Y Diet is essential before, during and following stress. In addition, many of the real foods in this diet plan curb the stress response or protect tissues from damage caused by cortisol. For example,

- A G-Spot snack, rich in whole grains, provides quality carbs to fuel brainpower and raises serotonin levels, which helps you calm down and cope. *(See page 17.)*

- Vitamin C–rich foods, such as citrus, red bell peppers and kiwi, help reduce blood pressure and cortisol levels.

- Seafood rich in the omega-3 fats help prevent the buildup of stress hormones.

- The healthy fats in nuts, seeds, olives and avocado discourage belly fat storage.

- The magnesium in legumes and dark green leafies helps curb the stress response, so you remain calmer in the face of stress.

- Crunchy foods, such as carrots, celery or jicama relieve tension in the jaw by giving you something to munch. Choose foods that take at least a minute to eat (as opposed to chips!).

- A little honey added to foods, such as a G-Spot snack of a toasted whole-grain English muffin drizzled with honey, improves memory and reduces anxiety.

Go with the Flow

The final piece of think-your-way-to-sexy is to keep blood flowing freely and smoothly to and from the brain. Let's face it. Sex is all about circuitry and circulation. Keep the nerve cells in tip-top shape, and make sure they have an unhindered supply of oxygen- and nutrient-rich blood, then sit back and enjoy life in your sexy skin.

Healthy and smooth blood vessels are built from a diet based on fiber-rich fruits and vegetables, whole grains, legumes and nuts, and low in artery-clogging saturated fats from red meats, fatty dairy products and processed or fast foods. That's the same eating plan that will help you cut inches off the waistline, which further improves the elasticity and smoothness of your vessels.

The B vitamins are especially important in keeping arteries clear and inflammation at bay. They block formation of a compound called homocysteine, which irritates blood vessels and initiates inflammation. Amp up intake of vitamins B_6 and B_{12}, as well as folic acid, and homocysteine doesn't stand a chance.

These vitamins are also important in making brain chemicals, such as serotonin, in generating energy for the brain and in maintaining healthy brain cells. With age or with the use of antacids, the body is less efficient at absorbing vitamin B_{12}. Up to one in every two seniors is deficient in this vitamin, with the first symptom being memory loss. Lana, a 42-year-old flight attendant I met on a flight from New York told me she had gotten to the point where she couldn't remember anything from one moment to another. "I thought for sure it was Alzheimer's," she told me. But a lab test found that Lana's memory lapses were a result of low vitamin B_{12}. "No one told me that the medication I was taking for heartburn would block absorption of this vitamin. All it took was a supplement twice daily, and my memory came back stronger than ever!"

Both folic acid and vitamin B_{12} are better absorbed from supplements than from food, so hedge your bets and get these nutrients from both.

- Vitamin B$_6$: bananas, seafood and whole grains, and 5 milligrams in a multi.
- Vitamin B$_{12}$: chicken breast, plain yogurt and fortified soymilk, and 25 micrograms in a multi.
- Folic acid: green leafies, legumes and orange juice, and 400 micrograms in a multi.

Of course, all the 40+ nutrients your body needs to grow, rejuvenate and repair are also essential to the brain and bloodstream. Most important is supplying them in the right balance. Too much of one nutrient and not enough of another can backfire, resulting in memory loss. That explains why people who follow the S-Ex-Y Diet and take a well-balanced multivitamin and -mineral also perform the best on tests for memory, learning, reaction times and problem solving.

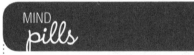

MIND *pills*

There are supplements that promise to boost memory. Do they work?

Omega-3 DHA: Improves memory, mind and mood. Suggested dose: 220–900 milligrams daily.

Phosphatidyl Serine (PS): Might improve learning, memory and recall (of names, faces, numbers, etc.) up to 30%. Start with a daily dose of 300 milligrams then drop that to a 100-milligram maintenance dose after a few weeks.

Ginkgo Biloba: Improves circulation and might help protect the hippocampus from damage and shrinkage. It is also an antioxidant. Suggested dose: 90 milligrams daily, with at least 24% flavone glycosides.

Lecithin: Contains choline, a component of the memory-enhancing nerve chemical acetylcholine. Pharmaceutical-grade lecithin improves memory, while studies are mixed on whether regular supplements are beneficial. Supplements on the market contain anywhere from 20–90% choline. A typical daily dose is 2,500–3,000 milligrams, four times a day. Or take a choline supplement of 250–500 milligrams daily.

Huperzine A: Might help block the breakdown of acetylcholine, and help Alzheimer's patients. Typical dose: 50–200 micrograms daily.

Acetyl-L-Carnitine (ALC): Chemically similar to choline and might aid memory, blood flow, sperm mobility and energy level. Suggested dose: 1,500–2,000 milligrams daily.

Tyrosine: An amino acid and building block for nerve chemicals, such as dopamine. Might prevent decline in cognition, especially associated with stress. Suggested dose: 100 milligrams/kg body weight, or 6,800 milligrams for a 150-pound person.

For example, other B vitamins and vitamins D, K, C, E and A improve concrete and abstract thinking, and lower the risk for dementia. Minerals such as iodine, chromium, boron, selenium, iron, copper and zinc improve concentration, learning skills, memory and overall brain function.

Jog Your Brain

Are you truly serious about staying mentally sharp? Then there are no excuses! You must exercise daily—both muscles and brain. People who challenge their brains by learning, problem solving and trying new things, and who exercise every day, also think faster, remember more, learn more easily, and are more creative and better problem solvers. They are least likely to develop memory loss, dementia or Alzheimer's. They also have more energy, motivation and desire to learn. They are happier, more content with their lives and more optimistic. In short, they feel confident, energized and sexy. *(See Chapters 9 and 10.)*

Makes sense. Mental stimulation increases the number of nerve connections in the brain, while exercise improves blood flow to the brain, which means more oxygen and nutrients. Activity raises levels of the feel-good nerve chemicals, the endorphins, and the get-moving nerve chemical, norepinephrine, which is associated with improved memory storage and retrieval. It boosts the body's production of brain-derived nerve growth factor (BDNF), a substance that keeps neurons strong and raises levels of neurophins that increase growth and connections between nerve cells. Both mental and physical exercise slow brain aging and sharpen mental function, reverse some memory loss, lift spirits and help the brain multitask. In fact, you will cut your risk for dementia by half if you exercise daily. Moderate exercise, such as brisk walking, will maintain your brain. Intense exercise, where you push your limits, actually regrows brain tissue. *(See Chapter 9.)*

From Brain Dead to Brain Trust

I can't think of one reason why any one of us would want to neglect our brain. All it takes is the S-Ex-Y Diet, daily exercise, a few good supplements and a stimulating life, and you stack the deck in favor of being one sharp cookie well into your 90s!

4

TAKE IT OFF
take it all off

THE PROMISE

Within ONE WEEK of making these changes, you will

- ✓ Lose at least 2 pounds.
- ✓ Have a sense of how easy it is to incorporate weight-management diet tricks into your lifestyle.

In SIX MONTHS, you will

- ✓ Have lost up to 50 pounds.
- ✓ Feel more confident.
- ✓ Need to purchase new, smaller-sized clothes.
- ✓ Have lowered your risk for all age-related diseases, from heart disease to sexual dysfunction.

In 20 YEARS, you will

- ✓ Have maintained the weight loss.
- ✓ Enjoy a vibrant life and an active sex life.
- ✓ Have increased your chances of outliving and outremembering your overweight friends.

Sexy comes in all shapes and sizes. Tanya felt sexiest, most confident, vibrant and sultry when she was skinny. Lana felt her best when she was a bit curvy and plump. Jim feels best when he works out at the gym every day and likes his lovers with abs of steel, but Tom prefers a soft tummy and ample hips, and his wife likes her man with a little extra padding around the middle. Whatever size and shape make you feel most comfortable and at ease in your own skin, that's the figure for you.

But let's get real here. Almost 7 out of 10 of us are too heavy; 1 in 3 is downright obese. If a shape isn't good for your mood, mind, heart or health, then it won't be sexy, either. Period. Your sexy self is your healthy self.

The goal is to get honest—brutally honest—about what you look like. That means accepting the imperfections that make you unique, but also identifying what needs changing and how fast.

Stop It. You're Killin' Me

Fat isn't sexy if it's killing you. Being overweight increases your chances of developing breast cancer, prostate cancer, endometrial cancer, lung cancer and just about every other cancer. It radically ups your risk for heart disease, high blood pressure, type 2 diabetes, stroke, asthma, sleep apnea, arthritis, gallbladder disease, menstrual problems and gout. Fat deposited around the middle is especially harmful, since it is biologically active, secreting inflammatory chemicals, dumping fat fragments into the blood and altering insulin levels, all of which make you sick and shorten your life.

There's a catch-22 issue to mood and figure, too. Being overweight increases the risk of depression, sleep disorders and fatigue, which causes overeating and more weight gain, which further depresses your mood. Studies show that anger and hostility escalate as a person's waistline expands, while self-esteem plummets. All that cranky is just one more reason why overweight people are much less likely to date than their fitter, leaner friends.

Weight gain hijacks life. Lugging around an extra 20, 40 or 200 pounds is exhausting, which leaves less energy to fully engage in living. The constant internal dialogue surrounding weight crowds out positive thoughts of planning the next adventure, remodel, class or shopping spree. It taints everything by painting it with a cloud of anxiety. How many minutes, hours, days, years, decades have people wasted thinking about their weight!? All that talk and no action makes Jane a very dull girl! Besides, would you want your tombstone to read: Dedicated my life to worrying about body fat?

Weight wreaks havoc with a person's sex life. Excess body fat acts as an endocrine gland pumping out the hormone estrogen, which increases breast cancer risk and lowers sex drive. In men, excess fat boosts the secretion of an enzyme called aromatase that converts testosterone into estradiol, a form of estrogen. This increases prostate cancer risk and lowers testosterone levels, leaving a man feeling tired, flabby and less interested in sex. It also reduces sperm count, gives him "man boobs," and leads to erectile dysfunction (ED). In fact, overweight men have up to a 90% greater risk for ED than do lean or fit men. Even the medications to treat obesity-related diseases, such as beta blockers or diabetes meds, increase weight gain in men and women and ED in men.

Every single one of these physical, emotional and sexual problems vanishes with weight loss.

What is Your Happy Weight?

Seven out of 10 people reading this sentence are overweight. Are you one of them? Do you know if you are?

Americans are in serious denial about their expanding waistlines. Being fat has become normal, so many people don't even realize they are overweight. In a Harris survey, people gave their heights and weights, which then were calculated to obtain body mass index (BMI) scores. A third of those in the overweight category thought they were normal size, while 70% of those classified as obese thought they were simply overweight. Interestingly, about half of obese people didn't think they were eating the wrong foods and only 27% of morbidly obese people said they ate more than they should. Are you kidding me?!!

Your happy weight should be your healthy weight, which is:

- **Body Mass Index (BMI):** A BMI of 24 or less. A BMI of 25 is overweight and 30+ is obese. For example, a 5'4" woman weighing at least 145 pounds, or a 5'10" man who weighs at least 174 pounds is overweight.

- **The Waist-to-Hip Ratio (WHR):** Wrap a measuring tape around your waist at its narrowest point. Measure your hips at the widest point. Then divide the waist measurement by the hip measurement. For women, a ratio less than 0.8 and for men a ratio of less than 1.0 is healthy. For example, a woman with a waist measurement of 32" and a hip measurement of 38" has a waist-to-hip ratio of 0.84—unhealthy. A man with waist and hip measurements of 37" and 40", respectively, has a WHR of 0.93—OK.

- **Tape Measure:** Less than 35 inches around the waist for a woman and less than 40 inches for a man is healthy.

- **The Mirror Test:** Strip in front of a full-length mirror. Take a good look at yourself. Then jump up and down. Anything that jiggles is excess body fat. (Boobs are off limits for this test—they will jiggle no matter how skinny you are!)

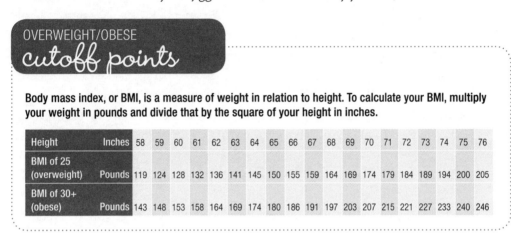

OVERWEIGHT/OBESE cutoff points

Body mass index, or BMI, is a measure of weight in relation to height. To calculate your BMI, multiply your weight in pounds and divide that by the square of your height in inches.

Height	Inches	58	59	60	61	62	63	64	65	66	67	68	69	70	71	72	73	74	75	76
BMI of 25 (overweight)	Pounds	119	124	128	132	136	141	145	150	155	159	164	169	174	179	184	189	194	200	205
BMI of 30+ (obese)	Pounds	143	148	153	158	164	169	174	180	186	191	197	203	207	215	221	227	233	240	246

Fruit From the Garden of Good and Evil

Body shape tells a lot about a person's health. Apple-shaped people carry most of their weight in the chest and abdomen, while pear-shaped people store fat below the belt and remain relatively slender in their upper bodies. A man with a waist of 40 inches and a woman with a waist of 35 inches or greater is likely to be an Apple.

Apples are more likely to develop heart disease, diabetes, depression, dementia, high blood pressure, erectile dysfunction, low sex drive and gallbladder disease; their diseases progress faster and more seriously; and they are more apt to die prematurely from disease than are Pears, even when the two have similar body weights and body fat percentages. In addition, blood cholesterol and triglyceride levels are high in Apples, while good cholesterol—HDL cholesterol—is low. Apples are 15 times more likely to develop endometrial cancer and are at higher risk for breast cancer than are pear-shaped women. The health risks apply to both slim and plump Apples.

The type of abdominal fat associated with health risks is called *visceral fat,* the firm fat that surrounds internal organs. Subcutaneous fat that lies close to the skin is not the culprit. So a firm, big belly is more indicative of health problems, while an inch of pinchable fat around the middle might force you to loosen your belt, but it probably won't hurt your health.

Why should middle fat affect health differently than hip fat? Fat above the waist is more saturated (firmer) than fat below the waist. It also is more metabolically active. It releases its fat into the blood, and interferes with blood sugar and fat regulation. Upper body fat also increases estrogen and lowers testosterone levels, which elevate the risk for cancer and lowers sex drive.

The good news is that visceral fat is the easiest to lose. Drop 10% of your body weight and you reduce abdominal fat by up to 30%. You'll also feel sexier and reduce your risk for most diseases. Teresa, an investment banker in Denver, had failed at a dozen different diets. "I had this all-or-nothing attitude about my weight. When I couldn't get to my ideal, I threw in the towel. I finally decided to give myself a little wiggle room and settle on a weight that was easier to maintain. I found I was not only happier, but hotter. Well, at least that's what my husband says!"

Don't get me wrong—obesity is still a health risk, regardless of body shape. It's just that the health danger escalates when that fat is packed around the middle.

Diets are for Super Dummies

The #1 stupidest weight-loss habit (other than taking up smoking…but that is over-the-top stupid) is to jump on a fad diet bandwagon. Diets don't work. In case you didn't hear me, let me say it again: FAD DIETS DEFINITELY DO NOT—UNDER ANY CIRCUMSTANCE—WORK.

I've been in the nutrition field for almost 30 years. I've seen hundreds of diets come and go. A few get recycled every decade or so. Never has one of them worked. The more they promise and the faster the weight loss, the more of a joke they are. Americans are fatter today than they were in the 1970s. That's because DIETS DON'T WORK!!!

You want to lose the weight, and for good. Yo-yo dieting leads to a metabolic slowdown. Repeated bouts of weight loss and gain increase abdominal fat, even when body weight remains the same. Fat is less metabolically active than muscle, so metabolism slows and it becomes increasingly more difficult to lose the unwanted pounds. Take Lily, for an example, who dropped from 145 pounds to 125 pounds and lost 15 pounds of fat and 5 pounds of muscle. When she regained the weight, she gained 18 pounds of fat and only 2 pounds of muscle. She was fatter as a result of dieting and gained more fat above the waist, even though her weight remained constant.

To maintain a desirable figure takes a lifelong plan, not a "get in, drop a few pounds, and get out" diet. The fact that overweight people average more than four dieting attempts every year attests to the fact that many people choose the quick fix, not the solution. To feel comfortable in your skin and attain and maintain the best sexy shape for you means making changes that last a lifetime.

Take it off for Good

> ❝ *The big difference between those who keep the weight off and those who don't is that successes stop drawing a line between dieting and their normal lives.* ❞

Like the multitudes of weight-loss successes, you can lose weight for good. The National Weight Control Registry (NWCR)—an ongoing project conducted by Brown University and the University of Colorado—is brimming with success stories from people who have maintained a 60-pounds-or-more weight loss for at least five years. The registry and lots of other studies show that successful dieters are no different than you and me. Like most dieters, they spent years at the win-lose weight game before they finally were successful. Many were overweight as children, have one or more overweight parents or have gained weight gradually over time or after pregnancy. Why do they succeed when the rest fail? The answer is simple: They prepare themselves for the after-the-diet phase, while the diet duds don't.

Following the S-Ex-Y Diet guidelines is the best way to lose weight, and eases the transition to permanent weight loss. But, first, it takes commitment. You have to really want to change. Not because your 20-year high school reunion is coming up or your lover says you should, but because you really want to be confident, sexy, in charge or your body and your life. You really want to be vibrant.

The big difference between those who keep the weight off and those who don't is that successes stop drawing a line between dieting and their normal lives. They are committed to revising their lives for good, adopting weight-loss strategies based on the S-Ex-Y Diet that become permanent habits.

The 12 Super-Sexy, Foolproof Tricks for Permanent Weight Loss

When it comes to dieting, food isn't the issue—it's only the symptom of a deeper need. Food stops serving the role of nurturer, companion or entertainment when people learn to nurture themselves and set realistic limits. As a result, their lives work better and they no longer need to overeat. It is not just a matter of eating less. If you're serious about reaching and sustaining a realistic weight, then *Commitment* becomes your middle name.

Donna, a legal secretary in Chicago, had a history of repeated failed dieting attempts. What made the difference the last time was her commitment to change, including decisions to permanently change the way she ate and thought, how much she moved and how well she organized her life, problem-solved and strategized. "I had to take a hard look at the role food played in my life. When I did that, I found I was using food to calm myself down and soothe my anger. I chose to use exercise to do that instead and I've lost 35 pounds and have kept it off for the past seven years!"

The tried-and-true, foolproof skills to lose weight and keep it off can be summarized in the 12-Step S-Ex-Y Weight Loss Plan that follows.

Foolproof Trick #1: Be a Planner

There's a saying that "Failing to plan is planning to fail." Nowhere does that apply more than with permanent weight loss. Amber, a stay-at-home mom in New Orleans, has maintained a 25-pound weight loss for six years. She started her plan by setting realistic expectations and limits on herself. "I asked myself, 'Is this reasonable for me at this time in my life?' When the answer to that question was a firm 'yes,' then I started to change my eating and exercise habits."

Like Amber, you'll need to plan your meals, your daily exercise and how you will handle personal high-risk situations from stress, parties and travel to eating in restaurants and boredom. Anticipate problems and go into battle well-armed with a plan. Even have a plan for when you slip up. Leave little to chance. Watch your weight, self-monitor your eating and exercise habits, and have backup plans for how you'll handle problem situations. "What really helped me was putting aside the idea of dramatic weight loss. Instead, I set a goal to lose about 2 pounds a week, which gave me some wiggle room," says Amber.

Foolproof Trick #2: Stay Alert

Monitor your progress. All those I know who lost weight for good have kept a food journal in which they recorded what, how much, when and where they ate, as well as hunger level and mood before and after the meal. This fosters self-awareness, keeps you focused on your goals, provides invaluable feedback and is a critical step in designing strategies.

Pay attention to your needs. Check your feelings frequently throughout the day by asking yourself, "How do I feel?" and "What do I need?" Keep close track of your daily exercise and weight. Jot down how much time is spent sitting or lying down to help motivate yourself to exercise. Place a mirror in the dining room. People eat less when they can see themselves eating!

Be honest, specific and complete in your record keeping. (Diet successes are consistently more accurate about portion size than are diet failures.) Record information at mealtime, since memory is highly inaccurate. Return to record keeping at the first sign of weight gain.

Foolproof Trick #3: Shake It Baby, Shake It

The most important predictor of whether or not you will succeed at permanent weight loss is how much you exercise. While some studies recommend burning at least 1,500 calories a week exercising, the NWCR found that successful losers burn almost twice that, or about 2,800 calories,

WHAT'S A *kiss worth?*

Sex burns calories. The longer and wilder the romp, the more calories burned.

ACTION	CALORIES
Masturbation	100–150
Tickling	17
Swooning	6
Kissing (1 hour)	120–325
Unclasping bra with hands	8
one-handed	18
with mouth	87
Foreplay	30–400
Intercourse	50–100*
Orgasm	60–100

* Having sex three times a week burns up to 7,500 calories per year. That's the equivalent of jogging 75 miles. The more intense the sex, the more calories burned—up to 15,000 calories annually (if you're making love three times a week). Burning 15,000 calories amounts to more than 4 pounds of body fat loss per year!

which is the equivalent of walking 4 miles or taking 10,000 steps every day. Granted, they probably didn't start out at that level of exercise, but they gradually increased their activity so that by the time they were seasoned maintainers, they were very active.

While most maintainers buy a pedometer and walk for exercise or combine activities, such as aerobics or swimming, how you burn the calories doesn't seem to matter. Even taking the stairs or using a push lawn mower counts toward your daily quota.

Foolproof Trick #4: Follow the S-Ex-Y Diet Guidelines

You will be most successful at weight loss if you follow the S-Ex-Y Diet guidelines, which means lots of vegetables, fruits, whole grains, legumes, nuts and other authentic food. Also watch calories and fat intake. Once you've lost the weight, you can be just a little freer with your choices.

How free can you be? First, lose the weight with a calorie quota of about 10 calories for every pound of desired body weight. If you want to weigh 135 pounds, that would mean 1,350 calories for basic living. Add an additional 5 calories/pound on the days you exercise for at least 45 minutes (for a total of 2,025 calories). Once you've lost the weight, add 100 calories each week to your daily weight-loss plan until your weight stabilizes.

SPICE UP
your love life

Some yummy spices and herbs also could help with weight loss, reduce hunger, improve mood or boost brainpower.

- **Red pepper:** In one study, women who added 2 teaspoons of dried red pepper to their daily diet consumed fewer calories during meals, which helped them drop pounds.
- **Capsaicin:** The heat in chili peppers releases feel-good brain chemicals called endorphins, and burns up to 50 calories a day, the equivalent of a half-pound loss each month.
- **Rosemary:** The antioxidants in this herb protect delicate tissues throughout the body, from brain to sex organs.
- **Turmeric:** This spice reduces inflammation, helps muscles repair themselves, protects the brain from aging, breaks up abnormal proteins that cause plaque associated with Alzheimer's and improves heart health.
- **Saffron:** A dose twice a day might be as good as Prozac in lowering depression rates. Add to rice while cooking.
- **Cinnamon:** Speeds the rate at which the brain processes visual cues, helps regulate blood sugar and helps you stay focused.
- **Garlic:** Helps brain cells fend off cancer.

Foolproof Trick #5: Sip Sparingly

It is easy to drink away your waistline. Liquid calories don't fill us up, so they are calories added to a day's worth of eating, rather than substitutes for other calories. The typical American averages 54 gallons of soft drinks a year. That's 86,400 empty calories, or the equivalent of 25 pounds of body fat. The link between soda and weight gain is so strong that literally every ounce consumed in a week ups your risk for being overweight.

With alcohol, the calories add up even faster. Sip a Long Island iced tea and you've downed the calorie equivalent of a platter of French fried onion rings. Have two apple martinis and a glass of wine at Happy Hour and you gulped the calories in two Quarter Pounders! And, watch out for serving size. A pint-sized margarita is four servings and close to 800 calories. Besides, alcohol dissolves your resolve; one glass of wine and you're likely to throw the diet out the window and order the Buffalo wings.

Foolproof Trick #6: Be Serving Savvy

Almost everyone seriously underestimates what they eat, guessing they eat about 800 calories less than they actually do each day. (Over the course of a month, that is the fat equivalent of almost 7 pounds.) The heavier people are, the more they fudge the numbers. We overestimate our daily exercise and fruits/vegetables intake (no, the three blueberries in a muffin is NOT a serving!), but seriously underestimate how much refined grains and meat we eat. That's why S-Ex-Y Diet Guideline #5—Remember that size matters—is critical if you want to lose the extra pounds forever.

Some dishonesty is intentional, but much of it is just a simple matter of not knowing portions. For a week, get out the food scale, the measuring cups and spoons, and do your homework. A serving of

- Meat/chicken/fish is 3 ounces, or the size of a deck of cards.
- Cooked whole grains (rice, oatmeal, pasta) is ½ cup, or the size of a small fist.
- Fruit or vegetables is 1 cup raw, ½ cup cooked or canned, 6 ounces juice.
- Nuts is 1 ounce or 2 tablespoons nut butter, or the size of a 9-volt battery.
- Milk or yogurt is 1 cup, or the size of a baseball.
- Oil/butter is 1 teaspoon, or the size of a postage stamp.

Foolproof Trick #7: Seek Possibilities, Not Problems

People who succeed at weight loss are confronted with the same high-risk situations as their diet-challenged cohorts. The difference is that diet failures fall victim to the situation, while diet successes control these situations by creative problem solving. For example, the #1 predictor of relapse is emotional issues, such as stress. Sara, an assistant professor at a major university in the Midwest was a stress eater. She solved her problem and lost 15 pounds by mapping out her trouble-prone situations and coming up with effective solutions. "Now I plan my life, rather than letting it happen to me. I call ahead to ask if a restaurant serves low-fat foods, I bring fruit platters to parties and I pack my own lunches so I'm not tempted by the doughnuts at work."

From your diet records, you'll identify high-risk situations. Write them down and develop plans for handling these situations. Revise those plans as needed.

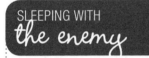

SLEEPING WITH
the enemy

Are you eating because you are truly hungry or is food a replacement for something else? The more "yes" answers you give to the following questions, the more likely it is that you are bedfellows with food, and that's the wrong lover!

1. Do you eat with a frenzy when under stress?

2. Do you constantly think about food and/or dieting?

3. Do you eat when you're bored, tired, lonely, depressed, anxious, scared or excited?

4. Do you eat to relax, as a reward or treat, or to calm down?

5. Does extra body weight give you a sense of self-protection?

6. Do you try to ignore hunger, but then feel deprived?

7. Are you driven by a desire to be "fit" or "thin" and believe that thinness is synonymous with success, beauty or personal power?

8. Do you overeat in secret or when you are alone?

9. Do you feel that physical hunger is more an enemy than a friend?

10. Do you eat unconsciously, that is, in front of the TV, while reading a book or magazine, or when preparing dinner?

Foolproof Trick #8: Get Selfish

Toss the "Good Girl"/"Nice Guy" syndrome. When you put others' needs before your own—like cooking what they prefer or trading exercise time to complete a project at work—you shove weight-management efforts to the back burner.

Instead, develop a healthy self-centeredness. Learn to identify how you feel and what you need, and you no longer will turn to food to feel emotionally satisfied. Call a friend if you are lonely, cry if you're sad, but eat only when you are physically hungry. This means taking care of, even pampering, yourself every day, including making daily exercise a #1 priority.

Foolproof Trick #9: Think Positive

What's on your mind is just as important as what's on your plate. Listen to your self-talk—those thoughts that repeat over and over again like a mantra. Allow only positive self-talk that will encourage and support your efforts. Replace negative internal messages ("I can't do this," "I'm no good") with positive supportive ones ("I'm making progress" or "I can do anything I set my mind to do!"). Have a firm conviction that you will succeed. Think of yourself as a person who takes control and is successful. That will improve your sex quotient, while boosting your weight-loss efforts.

Foolproof Trick #10: Put Together a Team

It's tough to stay on the diet track when everyone is eating chips and dip. You must convert sabotage into support to sustain your efforts through the tough times and to provide valuable feedback. Wherever possible, surround yourself with supportive family members and friends, or regularly attend a support group. Include loved ones in your new eating and exercise plans. Seek out successful role models, emulate them and ask them how they made healthy choices, started and stayed with exercise or boosted their self-esteem. Encouraging support takes two skills: asking for it and modeling it. Use assertive (not aggressive or passive) communication skills to ask specifically for the support you need from friends and family.

Foolproof Trick #11: Cut Yourself Some Slack

Give yourself permission to be imperfect. That means possibly settling for a heavier weight than you would like, but one that allows you a life, not a starvation routine.

Keep in mind that slips are normal and expected. The trick is not to let one day of missed exercise or an ice cream splurge undo your efforts. If you find yourself off track, pick up the pieces and start over again at the next meal or the next day.

Develop an early-warning plan to prevent slips from progressing to relapse. Reinstate record keeping, cut portions or exercise 10 extra minutes a day when your weight moves out of a 3- to 5-pound buffer zone. Remember: There are no mistakes, only feedback.

Foolproof Trick #12: Give Yourself Presents

> 66 Reach your goal by rewarding yourself every step of the way. 99

What will keep you motivated to stick with both a weight-loss plan and a weight-management life? What will sustain your determination? What are the benefits to finally saying "So long" to the diet roller coaster? Rewards and reinforcements, that's what. Jim, a bank teller in Columbia, South Carolina, found that when he rewarded himself, he was much more motivated to stay on track. "I created an ongoing list of nonfood bonuses for meeting my exercise and weight-loss goals. I was amazed how important those rewards became," he says. Those rewards might be clothing, a movie, quarters in a jar for every day you exercise (use the money to buy yourself new exercise equipment), a manicure or planting flowers.

In short, use the "if . . . then" rule. *If* you reach your goal, *then*, and only then, do you get the bonus. Reach your goal by rewarding yourself every step of the way.

20 WAYS TO
lose the blubber

1. **Make exercise fun.** Listen to books on tape, walk the dog, read a book on the Exercycle, vary your workouts with the season.

2. **Chew on this.** Eat two fruits and/or vegetables at every meal and one at every snack, and eat them first. You'll meet the 9-a-day quota, feel full and automatically cut back on calories.

3. **Take a hike, every hour.** Set the watch alarm on the hour and take a five-minute brisk walk around the office. Over the course of an eight-hour shift, you'll accrue 40 minutes of exercise. Stop using the kids as go-getters and throw out the remote, too!

4. **Brush your teeth after a meal.** This signals that you're finished eating and curbs cravings for dessert. Also, keep in mind: A craving is only a suggestion, it is not a command!

5. **Skip the boob tube.** Hours of television watching are directly proportional to weight gain. Go for an after-dinner walk, ride the exercise bike, do laundry or paint the living room instead. In fact, men who watch even 10 hours a week are twice as likely to develop erectile dysfunction compared to men who watch less, and 20% more likely than overweight men who don't watch TV.

6. **Eat with chopsticks.** You will eat slower and not shovel.

7. **Eat slowly.** This allows you to digest the food and gives the stomach time to tell the brain it's full.

8. **Drink first.** We often confuse thirst with hunger, diving for the ice cream when it's water our bodies need. Drink a glass of water and wait 15 minutes before giving in to a craving. You may find the hunger subsides.

9. **Challenge yourself.** If you're comfortable walking at a moderate pace, go up a short hill during your next walk or pick up the pace.

10. **Be a lark.** Exercise in the morning so you don't spend the rest of the day finding excuses why you can't exercise.

11. **Be an expert.** Learn to read labels and purchase mostly foods that contain no more than 3 grams of fat for every 100 calories (or approximately 30% fat calories).

12. **Doggie-bag it.** Most American restaurant servings are platters, not portions. Put half the serving in a doggie bag for tomorrow's lunch.

13. **Skip the fat-free/net-carb desserts.** Ounce for ounce, most fat-free desserts are just as calorie-dense as the higher-fat versions. Even if they are low-calorie, you aren't doing yourself any favors by eating the whole box. Stick to the serving size on the label.

14. **Eat less.** Cut your typical portions of everything except vegetables and fruit by one-quarter.

15. **Eat a salad or drink a glass of V8 juice before a meal.** You'll consume fewer calories.

16. **Flavor up.** Add herbs and spices, not oils and butter, to recipes.

17. **Calories count.** The 100 calories in a tablespoon of mayo on a sandwich equals 10½ pounds of excess body fat over one year.

18. **Eat soy.** A study from the University of Alabama found it reduces belly fat and aids in weight loss.

19. **Get enough sleep.** You're more likely to overeat and choose all the wrong foods (candy, chocolate, sugar and caffeine) when you're tired.

20. **Purchase a pedometer.** This small device is a great incentive to boost the number of steps you take every day.

Face the Battle of the Bite

Here is how to tweak the S-Ex-Y Diet to be healthier, happier and sexier:

1 **Lose weight gradually.** You want an eating plan you can live with for life and that will allow a gradual weight loss of 1 to 2 pounds a week. Strive for no less than 1,300 calories if you are short or relatively inactive (add an additional 500 calories if you are tall and/or active). You should increase exercise, not cut calories further, if you can't lose weight on this low-calorie plan. Also, you want to cut calories, not vitamins and minerals. That means making every bite count. Don't waste precious calories on foods high in sugar, refined grains and fat, and low in nutrients. Hey, would you pay to breathe in carbon monoxide? Of course not. Well, don't pay to eat junk!

> **66** When *is as important as* what *you eat.* **99**

2 **Focus on plants.** Most antioxidant-rich foods in the S-Ex-Y Diet—from fruits, vegetables and whole grains to nuts and legumes—are low in calories and high in fiber, which fill you up. Load the plate and base your snacks on these. Complement those foods with moderate amounts of calcium-rich foods (nonfat milk) and iron-rich foods (extra-lean meats, chicken or fish). Take a moderate-dose, well-balanced vitamin and mineral supplement to fill in any nutrient gaps.

3 **Eat frequently.** *When* is as important as *what* you eat. Large, infrequent meals might set up a feast-or-famine scenario whereby the body stores more calories as fat as a safeguard against what it perceives as a famine. By contrast, dividing the same amount of calories into five or more little meals and snacks encourages the body to "burn" the food for immediate energy rather than store it in the hips and thighs.

4 **Commit to health.** The ultimate goal is not just a certain figure or a number on the scale, it is a lifelong promise to yourself to strive to be your sexiest and healthiest. It is a lifetime commitment, not just to lose weight and keep it off, but to modify habits so they support health and, ultimately, maintain the best and sexiest weight for you.

Lose It, Lover

You can drop the extra pounds. I have no doubt. But you won't do it until you make the commitment. Then it's a matter of cutting back on junk food and moving your body the way it was designed to move. The more junk you cut and the more you move, the more weight you will lose. It's as simple as that.

5

ARE YOU
a looker?

THE PROMISE

Within TWO WEEKS of making these changes, you will

- ✓ Notice improvements in the color and glow of your skin.
- ✓ See changes as dry skin becomes more subtle.

In **SIX MONTHS**, you will

- ✓ Look younger.
- ✓ Have hair and nails that are stronger and healthier.
- ✓ Have lowered your risk for skin cancer and future wrinkling.
- ✓ Notice a reduction in fine lines and wrinkles.

In **20 YEARS**, you will

- ✓ Look up to 15 years younger than your age.

Connie and Lorraine are both in their 50s. Connie spends about $1,000 a month on cosmetics, haircuts, face cream, facials and what she calls "other beauty essentials." She spends even more on clothes, shoes and accessories, as well as diet books, pills, powders and shakes in hopes of dropping the accumulating inches around her waist and looking younger. She lives on packaged food from the diet center. Yet she can't keep the weight off and looks older than her years.

Lorraine, on the other hand, spends less than 10 minutes primping in the morning. She is careful about what she wears, but not obsessive, and spends her free time not at the spa, but at the local farmers' market. Her skin glows, her hair is shiny and carefree, and she radiates a beauty that makes heads turn wherever she goes. She's gained and lost a few pounds over the years, but has settled into a comfortable, healthy weight since menopause. She definitely would be classified as fit and trim. People often guess her to be up to 15 years younger than she is.

You might be thinking that Lorraine has all the luck. Probably born into a family with great genes, destined to be effortlessly gorgeous. You're wrong. Connie and Lorraine are identical twins.

I met Lorraine on a flight from New Jersey to Portland, Oregon. We talked about her diet and lifestyle, as well as her sister's struggles with beauty and weight. "She just doesn't get it," Lorraine said. "I've been telling her for years to take care of her inside and the outside will take care of itself." I couldn't have said it better.

Eat, Drink and be Pretty

Beauty is not skin deep, as the old adage suggests. Your skin, hair and outer appearance directly reflect your inner, deeper health. When your insides are glowing, so are your outsides.

> 66 There is nothing that makes its way more directly to the soul than beauty. 99
> —Joseph Addison

If you don't believe me, take a look around the grocery store. People look just like their shopping carts. A cart packed with Ding Dongs, Ho Hos, Cheez Whiz, chips, soft drinks, beer, white bread, candy and other processed junk is typically pushed by someone battling a weight problem and with dry, dull, lifeless skin and hair. People with radiant skin, shiny hair, a sexy figure, great posture and a twinkle in their eyes will be the ones with carts loaded with foods you'd find in the S-Ex-Y Diet. If Connie had spent as much time nourishing her skin from within as she spent on products rubbed on the outside of her body, she would look and feel as young as her twin sister.

Skin Essentials

> **"** *Beauty is not caused. It is.* **"**
> —Emily Dickinson

Skin is the body's biggest—and most visible—organ. It makes up 15% of your desirable body weight, and is composed of three layers: the subcutaneous, the corium (dermis) and the outer epidermis (the layer you see in the mirror). The subcutaneous layer is the deepest layer and consists of a resilient cushion of fat and collagen. (Skinfold calipers pinch this layer of fat to assess the percentage of overall body fat.)

The middle layer, called the corium or dermis, is the "true" skin. This layer contains both collagen and elastic fibers, and shields the subcutaneous layer from injury, while helping repair surrounding layers when they are damaged. An abundance of blood vessels and nerve endings provide oxygen and nutrients to this layer and the hair shafts and oil glands embedded here. Wrinkles originate in the corium.

The epidermis, or outer layer of the skin, is the thinnest layer. At the base of the epidermis, where it meets the corium, new cells are produced that move upward as dead cells are sloughed off and lost daily. Specialized cells in the epidermis manufacture skin pigment, provide immune defenses against infection and disease, and produce a protective protein called keratin that forms a physical barrier against chemicals, germs and other foreign substances.

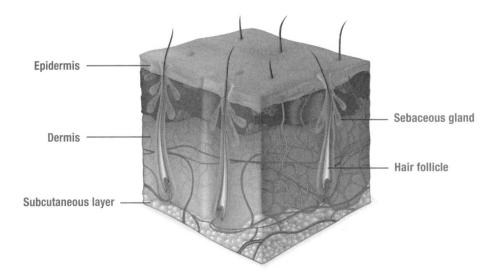

Epidermis

Sebaceous gland

Dermis

Hair follicle

Subcutaneous layer

All three layers of the skin are dependent on both diet and lifestyle. Skin mirrors the abuse you inflict on it when you eat junk, drink too much alcohol or caffeinated beverages, seldom get around to exercise, have chronic stress and sleep fitfully. Get smart and follow the S-Ex-Y Diet guidelines, drink plenty of water, move a lot, calm down and sleep well, and lo and behold, beauty experts will want you as their poster child!

What's Food Got to Do with It?

Food is loaded with skin essentials. From the water in a slice of watermelon to the amount of vitamin C in an orange, every one of the 40+ nutrients and the almost 1 million phytonutrients is critical to your looks. In addition, the top layer of the skin regenerates every month, so nutrient deficiencies, as well as optimal nutrient intake, show up very fast.

I'm not talking about really bad diets and major nutrient deficiencies. Granted, an absolutely awful diet will result in classic deficiency symptoms, such as beriberi, scurvy or pellagra, all of which cause some pretty gross skin problems. But you don't have to be so deficient in vitamin C that you develop scurvy with bleeding gums and tons of bruises, nor must you be so low in vitamin B_1 that your skin breaks out in a terrible rash from beriberi. Even slightly low intakes of one or more nutrients will have subtle, yet telltale, effects on complexion, the sparkle in your eyes or the sexy bounce of your hair.

Feeding the Whole Package

Everything I've told you so far about how what you eat affects energy, mood, sleep, ability to handle stress and weight also applies to how attractive

> 66 *Good looks is the outer glow of inner happiness.* 99

you are. That's because beauty is health. Good looks is the outer glow of inner happiness. When you are healthy, it shows. While depression saps the sparkle from your eyes, fatigue drains the glow from your cheeks and chronic stress causes your hair to go drab and fall out, happiness and health are sexy radiating from every pore. Feeling and being sexy isn't about how young, sleek or even fashionable you are. It's about an inner glow.

The good news is that the S-Ex-Y Diet boosts your appeal factor in every way. Follow the guidelines I've laid out in this book and you will improve your sexy self, from your mood, mind and complexion at the top of your head to the nails on the tips of your toes and every cell in between. The S-Ex-Y Diet feeds the whole package.

Camille said it best: "Within a few weeks of following Elizabeth's advice, I noticed that my skin and hair were healthier. I look more vibrant, which definitely makes me feel more secure in who I am. What a contrast to some of the women I work with, who have gained weight with each passing year. They struggle with basic things like walking and even standing. They don't act or look happy or healthy. While they are aging, I seem to get younger. I am determined to get better with age, and so far I'm doing pretty well!"

Eat right and you'll look great. Better yet, according to a study published in the *Journal of Sex Medicine,* women who are happy with themselves and feel good about how they look, are more easily aroused and have more orgasms than do women who haven't gotten with the sexy-self program.

Skin: From A to Zinc

> 66 *There is no cosmetic for beauty like happiness.* 99
> —Countess of Blessington

Every bite you take makes or breaks your skin. Nutrients from food make up the structure of skin, build a healthy blood supply to nourish skin, provide protection against sunlight and other damaging environmental onslaughts, help reduce disease and inflammation and jump-start the repair process when skin is hurt. For example,

- Water makes up 70% of skin, and helps flush out toxins, absorb nutrients and speed cell turnover and repair. The water you drink from a glass or from that Quickie snack of watermelon plumps up skin cells, making them moist. Too little water and your skin is dry, flaky and drawn.

- Protein comprises 25% of skin. It builds supporting structures in the skin, such as collagen, that keep skin firm, elastic and resilient. Too little protein and your skin is dry, flaky and ages rapidly.

- Healthy fats in salmon and olive oil comprise 5% of skin and ensure that it remains lubricated and moist.

- Every vitamin and mineral, from vitamin A to zinc, helps build, maintain protect skin from aging, damage and diseases such as cancer. *(See "The Skinny Nutrients," below.)*

Sexy is all about circulation, which is the skin's mass transit system, supplying building blocks to and removing toxins from every cell. Nutrients essential to the maintenance of red blood cells (the oxygen carriers in the blood) include protein, iron, folic acid and other B vitamins, copper, vitamin C, selenium and vitamin E. Skimp on any of these nutrients and you cut off the skin's supply of oxygen and nutrients, while allowing toxic waste products to accumulate. The skin becomes sallow, dry, pale and lifeless when even one of these nutrients is in short supply. Beyond skin, poor circulation leaves you feeling frumpy, dull and lifeless, which is about as sexy as a flat tire!

THE SKINNY ON
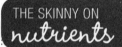

All nutrients are related to healthy skin. Here are a few examples why, and what foods you need to maintain a healthy glow.

Nutrient	The Skin Connection	Foods in the S-Ex-Y Diet
Water	Maintains skin moisture; helps maintain normal oil secretion.	Water, fresh fruit, tea
Protein	Maintains underlying muscles and skin structure, elasticity, resiliency; maintains hormones that regulate skin moisture; regulates skin pigments.	Low-fat milk, meat, fish, chicken, legumes
Good Fats	Maintain skin moisture. Deficiency results in scaly, dry skin. Omega-3s reduce inflammation & wrinkling; improve elasticity and wound healing.	Safflower oil, nuts, seeds, whole grains, fatty fish, DHA-fortified foods
Vitamin A	Maintains outer layer of skin; (beta-carotene) protects against skin cancer and premature aging.	Dark green/orange veggies and fruits
Vitamin D	Protects against sun damage.	Fortified milk, soymilk, orange juice
Vitamin E	Antioxidant that helps prevent premature aging and skin cancer.	Nuts, seeds, wheat germ

Continued

Nutrient	The Skin Connection	Foods in the S-Ex-Y Diet
Vitamin K	Might lighten under-eye circles, aids circulation.	Dark green leafy veggies
Vitamin B$_2$	Deficiency causes blisters and cracks at the corner of the mouth, oily and flaky skin.	Low-fat milk, dark green veggies, mushrooms
Niacin	Deficiency causes dermatitis. Helps skin cells use energy optimally.	Chicken breast, peanut butter, green peas
Vitamin B$_6$	Deficiency causes itching, dry skin; anemia. Helps build proteins.	Bananas, lean meat, fish, chicken breast
Folic Acid	Deficiency causes anemia; pale skin. Helps cells regenerate.	Dark green veggies, orange juice, legumes
Vitamin B$_{12}$	Deficiency causes anemia; pale skin.	Low-fat milk, lean meat, fish, chicken breast
Pantothenic Acid	Deficiency causes dry, flaky skin.	Low-fat milk, chicken breast, peanut butter, veggies, brown rice
Vitamin C	Maintains oil-producing glands, collagen, skin elasticity and resiliency; antioxidant that helps prevent premature aging and skin cancer.	Citrus fruits, red bell peppers, kiwi, strawberries
Copper	Prevents anemia, protects skin cells.	Oysters, avocado, fish, soy
Iron	Prevents anemia, dark circles under the eyes; improves blood flow to the skin.	Dark green veggies, lean red meat, legumes, dried fruit
Selenium	Antioxidant that helps prevent skin cancer.	Organ meats, seafood, whole grains
Zinc	Maintains collagen and elastin; might prevent stretch marks; helps heal cuts & treat acne; deficiency causes dry, rough skin.	Oysters, turkey breast, wheat germ, whole grains
Glutathione	Protects skin from damage.	Peaches, asparagus, cabbage, cauliflower
Lycopene	Reduces skin redness and skin cancer.	Tomatoes, watermelon
Polyphenols	Reduce skin cancer, wrinkling.	Tea, chocolate, berries
Anthocyanins	Reduce skin cancer.	Berries, grape seed
Terpenes	Reduce skin cancer.	Citrus fruits

Skin Loves an Orgy

> 66 *The real sin against life is to abuse and destroy beauty, even one's own—even more, one's own, for that has been put in our care and we are responsible for its well-being.* 99
>
> —Katherine Anne Porter

Age is not the skin's public enemy #1. Sunlight is. Ultraviolet (UV) rays in sunlight generate oxygen fragments called free radicals. These highly reactive compounds pierce delicate cell membranes and attack the genetic code within skin cells, damaging underlying structures, such as collagen and elastic fibers.

The genetic code within each skin cell suffers thousands of free-radical hits every day, or up to 4 ¼ pounds of free radicals in a year (even more when we are sick or unhealthy). UVA light penetrates the outer layers of the skin, causing sunburn, sun spots, rough texture and skin cancer. UVB light penetrates deeper skin layers, causing wrinkles. Those UV rays damage skin on the ski slopes in winter and through cloud cover in the fall, just as easily as on the beach in the summer.

Fortunately, antioxidants protect skin and eyes from free-radical damage. Frequent sun exposure and smog both deplete antioxidants in these tissues. It also takes up to three months to accumulate antioxidants in skin. So you must front-load tissue stores by having an antioxidant orgy daily. These antioxidants work as a team, so a combination is better than focusing on just one or two.

Vitamin C is an important antioxidant defender. Sun exposure (as well as stress) drains this vitamin from the skin for up to 72 hours, leaving skin vulnerable to damage. Just a few hours of sun exposure also depletes vitamin E from the skin (by up to 50%!), while boosting intake of this antioxidant, alone or in combination with other antioxidants like beta-carotene, selenium and vitamin C, helps lower skin-cancer risk. Vitamin E also slows skin aging by reducing the production of an enzyme called collagenase that otherwise breaks down collagen, causing the skin to sag and wrinkle.

Beta-carotene accumulates in the skin, providing 24-hour antioxidant protection against sun damage. As little as ½ cup of cooked carrots every day provides enough beta-carotene to reduce the redness and skin inflammation of sunburn, a sign of accelerated aging and cancer risk. The more carotene-rich produce you eat, the more skin protection you get. (Oops: Eating too many carotene-rich foods, such as sweet potatoes, carrots and mangoes, can turn skin slightly orange, but this is harmless and doesn't show up at all with a light bottle tan.)

Don't forget to drink tea, too! Tea contains antioxidant compounds, called polyphenols, that reduce sun damage associated with wrinkling and cancer. Tea also reduces inflammation and redness associated with sunburn. While green tea is the best source of polyphenols, all kinds of tea, including black, red and white, contain these helpful compounds.

That's just the tip of the antioxidant iceberg. The almost 1 million phytonutrients in colorful fruits and vegetables, green tea, nuts, legumes and other real foods in the S-Ex-Y Diet are an orgy of antioxidants. For example, carotenoids in all colorful produce, alpha-lipoic acid in spinach, pycnogenol, glutathione, phytoestrogens in tofu and lycopene in watermelon reduce the risk of skin injury from sun exposure.

How much do you need? If you are really, truly, sincerely dedicated to looking your best, youngest and most vibrant, then you need to take S-Ex-Y Diet Guideline #1—Have an antioxidant orgy—very seriously. That's what Lorraine did. Shopping at the local farmers' market, she loaded up on colorful produce and made sure to include some at every meal. Like Lorraine, aim for at least nine servings of colorful fruits and vegetables every day. Mix it up, too. The best skin rejuvenation comes from a variety of produce, not bingeing on acai berry juice, goji bars or the current fruit-de-jour fad.

Take the Pill

You also might consider S-Ex-Y Diet Guideline #6—Take the pill. Some antioxidants are needed by skin in amounts difficult to get from food alone. Selenium, for example, is in abundant supply in foods grown on selenium-rich soil, but how do you know if your broccoli came from the right farm? To consume the minimum amount of vitamin E shown to protect skin would require eating 16 cups of almonds, 1 ½ cups of safflower oil or 124 cups of fresh spinach every day. Not likely!

Then there are some foods that are best in extract form. Grape seed extract (GSE), for example, is a great source of vitamin E, flavonoids, linoleic acid (a healthy fat that keeps skin moist) and antioxidants. This extract is rich in resveratrol, which helps cancer cells commit suicide before they cause trouble. As a result, GSE aids in skin healing, protects against skin cancer, provides some sunscreen protection, reduces edema and helps prevent wrinkling, inflammation and even skin infections. A safe dose is 50 to 100 milligrams in capsules or a few drops in water or tea.

Consider taking a moderate-dose multiple vitamin and mineral, along with extra antioxidants, such as 500 milligrams of vitamin C, 100 micrograms of selenium (as selenomethionine) and 100 IU of vitamin E (as d-alpha tocopherol). Other skin-loving supplements include glutathione (at a daily dosage of at least 100 milligrams/day along with extra vitamin C) and pycnogenol (start at 150–200 milligrams a day for two weeks, then cut back to 20–100 milligrams as a maintenance dose). (See Chapter 8.)

Rub It on Me!

Following the S-Ex-Y Diet and popping a few of the right supplements absolutely will make a difference in your appearance. Like Lorraine, you might look up to 15 years younger as a result.

However, antioxidants obtained from the diet are stored primarily in the deeper subcutaneous layer of the skin, thus leaving the corium and outer epidermis only partially protected. In short, the body delivers a certain amount of nutrients to the skin, no matter how much you eat or swallow. The solution? Give skin the ol' one-two punch by feeding it from the inside and rubbing nutrients on the outside.

Some nutrients in the right concentration can help turn back the clock and lower skin-cancer risk when applied topically. In one study, the forearms of volunteers were treated with vitamin C solutions or placebos and then were exposed to UV light. The sites treated with vitamin C showed significantly less sun damage, compared to the untreated group. Because damage continues for hours or days after sun exposure, applying vitamin C before and after sun exposure also might help prevent or repair long-term damage. Vitamin C solutions applied to the skin also might help fade liver spots and curb damage to underlying collagen, thus preventing wrinkles. Use the right formula and you boost the skin's vitamin C level by 40%.

Here's the catch. The lotion, cream, extract or serum must contain at least a 10% vitamin C concentration or it is useless. Also, vitamin C breaks down easily, especially in the presence of light. So purchase products in small, opaque bottles, and refrigerate them.

Vitamin E is another inny-and-outy vitamin. Applied topically, it acts as a mild sunscreen (i.e., SPF 3), reduces UV-induced skin damage even when applied after exposure and penetrates the skin's surface, preventing wrinkles. It must be supplied in at least a 1% solution, or it will do little more than drain your pocketbook.

Other antioxidants, such as beta-carotene, limonene, ergothionine and lycopene, rubbed into skin, boost immune responses that, in turn, protect against UVA damage. Vitamin K applied topically helps speed recovery and reduce redness from laser surgery, and might reduce under-eye circles (but must be applied religiously for at least four months before you'll notice a difference). Then there is aloe, which when applied to sunburned skin, helps reduce inflammation and redness associated with sunburn. Other topicals waiting in the wings include citronellol, rosmarinus officinalis, grape seed extract and evening primrose.

Then there are foods that also aid skin. Tea is my favorite skin lotion. Back in the days before sunscreen, my mother would make a pot of strong black tea, cool it down and pour it over me when I came home with a sunburn. It took the sting out of the burn and helped prevent peeling. Little did I know that, years later, scientists would discover that topical application of tea lowers skin damage from UV light, reduces inflammation and redness, strengthens the epidermis and even helps lower skin-cancer risk. Tea contains a batch of antioxidants, including quercetin, a flavonol that reduces free-radical damage to skin cells. One more reason to say, "Thanks, Mom!!"

Cucumbers are natural astringents and also reduce inflammation in the skin, which is just what the doctor ordered for tightening pours and soothing a mild sunburn or troublesome blemish. Cucumber juice has the same pH as the skin, so it is gentle even for delicate complexions. Also, cool cucumber slices placed over the eyes help reduce puffiness.

Honey has been used for centuries as an emollient, skin softener and cleanser. As a humectant, it also helps hold moisture in the skin. The tiny amounts of lactic acid in honey act as a gentle exfolient.

Oatmeal contains amino acids and oils that, when used in lotions and masks, help reduce itchy, dry skin and possibly reduce the discomfort from dermatitis, psoriasis, rashes and eczema. Or, rubbed directly on the skin, oats act as a gentle exfolient that scrub away dead skin.

Milk is so good for the skin, Cleopatra is said to have bathed in it. Applied directly to the skin, milk acts as a softener and moisturizer, probably because of its fats and proteins. It also is a great source of lactic acid, which helps sluff off dead skin cells, leaving the skin looking younger and softer.

Ginger can liven up skin, probably because of its ability to stimulate blood flow. Be careful; ginger can be irritating to some delicate complexions, so don't use it on your face.

Finally, papaya contains a protein-digesting enzyme called papain, which dissolves dead cells on the epidermis, while leaving the living, vibrant cells glowing. Mixed into a mask once a week, papaya is an inexpensive, all-natural alternative to expensive commercial masks.

By far the biggest nutritional bang for your buck comes from vitamin A (i.e., retinyl palmitate, retinyl linoleate, retinyl acetate or retinoic acid). This vitamin builds and maintains epithelial tissue, the linings of the body, including the skin. Apply vitamin A every night and you'll notice a huge improvement in acne, wrinkles, brown spots and you'll even out the texture and tone of your skin. It reduces pore size, increases the elastin fibers that give skin its bounce-back resiliency and even helps repair sun damage. It might cause flaking and itching for the first few months, but your skin will look years younger after that. I even rub it on the tops of my hands before bedtime.

Massage Oil

> 66 *You can take no credit for beauty at sixteen. But if you are beautiful at sixty, it will be your soul's own doing.* 99
>
> —Marie Carmichael Stopes

Fat is a tricky subject when it comes to skin. A low- to moderate-fat diet reduces the risk of skin cancer, prevents inflammation and stimulates the immune system to protect delicate skin cell membranes from damage, thus improving the skin's ability to defend itself from sunlight and aging. A bit of fat in the daily diet also ensures absorption of the fat-soluble vitamins A, D, E and K, all of which are essential for healthy skin. A few chunks of fatty avocado added to salsa, for example, boost absorption of antioxidants in the tomatoes 10-fold. But it's not just cutting back on fat. You must include the healthy fats in the S-Ex-Y Diet.

Anyone eating processed foods, fatty dairy products and greasy meat is asking for sallow skin, dull hair and skin cancer. The saturated and trans fats in these foods even increase the risk for balding in men, possibly because these fats damage hair follicles.

The worst combo is fat and sugar. Combined with refined grains, sugary foods and processed junk, bad fats fuel the fires of inflammation, an underlying cause of premature aging of the skin. Added sugars link to protein in the body, forming glycation end products (GEP) that age skin. Fat and sugar also increase the risk of

LOOK *busters*

Some habits are just plain bad for your looks. Here's what to do instead:

1. **Don't slouch.** In studies, people with bad posture are assumed to be dull, unsocial, unhealthy and less confident, while those who stand up straight are perceived as more attractive and intelligent, no matter what their body size, shape or age.

2. **Watch the booze.** Alcohol dehydrates the body, including the skin, and causes blood vessels at the skin's surface to leak, increasing the risk for puffiness, stretched skin, blotchy complexion and faster wrinkling. Limit alcohol to one drink a day, and make it red wine, if possible, since that has 20 times the skin-protecting antioxidants as white wine.

3. **Calm down.** It takes years for stress to ruin the heart and brain, but literally days to wreak havoc on skin and hair. Stress is a major factor in almost all skin disorders, from psoriasis to wrinkling. It reduces the skin's ability to defend itself against sun damage, dries the skin and makes it flaky, red and dull. It also can create the ultimate bad hair day with hair loss, dandruff, itchy scalp and oily hair.

4. **Get off your butt.** Sit on your duff and your skin semi-suffocates for oxygen. Exercise increases circulation, which makes skin and hair glow. It increases muscle tone that helps anchor and support skin. Exercisers also are happier, more energetic and invigorated, so they radiate a "come hither" energy that makes them attractive. Besides, people who exercise are thought to be years younger than their biological age.

5. **Avoid sunburn.** No matter how good the diet, you still must protect your skin, hair and eyes from sun damage. Use a broad-spectrum product rated SPF 15 or higher. Use it liberally and often. Choose a waterproof version if you are swimming or perspire heavily. Apply an SPF 15 lip balm, too. Wear a wide-brimmed hat and UV-blocking sunglasses.

6. **Stay cool to be hot.** Super-hot showers and baths, or using harsh soaps, dry the skin. Instead, take warm showers, moisturize afterwards and avoid bubble baths. Use rubber gloves when doing housework and always reapply lotion after washing your hands.

becoming overweight, which is another risk factor for bad complexion, premature aging of the skin and skin cancer. If you eat authentic 75% of the time, you automatically cut back on these skin-robbing foods. If you need something sweet, try xylitol. A sugar alcohol with half the calories, xylitol might help build skin collagen and reduce GEPs, thus helping age-proof skin.

On the other hand, fats that are good for your mood, mind, heart and body, also sexy-up your looks. The omega-3 fats make hair shiny, protect skin from sagging and wrinkling, speed healing, slow aging, and reduce skin-cancer risk. People who eat lots of S-Ex-Y foods—omega-3-rich seafood or foods fortified with an algal-based DHA, antioxidant-packed produce, nuts and olive oil—are also the ones with the fewest wrinkles. Salmon is a great source of skin-boosting omega-3s and it contains astaxanthin, an antioxidant that helps reduce inflammation and boost immunity in the skin. That's why S-Ex-Y Diet Guideline #4—Get wet and wild—is so important for your mirror image.

Eat Your Way to Sparkling Eyes

Years ago, people believed that the common causes of vision loss as we aged—cataracts and macular degeneration—were an inevitable consequence of getting older. Now we know

> 66 Of all the senses, sight must be the most delightful. 99
> —Helen Keller

there is much you can do to prevent, slow, stop and possibly even reverse this damage by making a few changes in what you eat today.

Long-term exposure to air and light generates oxidants that damage the eyes. The S-Ex-Y Diet, rich in antioxidant nutrients, such as vitamin C, vitamin E, selenium, beta-carotene, lutein and zinc, fortifies eyes against this damage. People with high levels of these antioxidants are at lowest risk of vision loss later in life. For example, when people consume as little as 10 milligrams of lutein daily (the amount found in ½ cup of spinach), their levels of lutein increase in the blood and eyes, and they are less prone to vision loss. If they do develop vision problems, the disease is less likely to progress to advanced stages.

Dietary fat might play a role in the development of age-related vision loss. Saturated fats in meat and fatty dairy products increase risk up to 80%, while the omega-3s in fatty fish lower risk for both cataracts and macular degeneration.

Those healthy fats also might help treat dry eyes, a condition characterized by itching, burning, irritation, redness, excessive tearing and blurred vision that only improves with blinking.

Sexy Smells

Being "a looker" goes beyond a glowing complexion, shiny hair and sparkling eyes. We also judge a potential partner by his or her smell, both consciously and unconsciously. No matter how handsome or pretty you are, if you stink, it's unlikely you'll be getting a second date.

Many of the foods in the S-Ex-Y Diet influence how luscious you smell. Researchers at Charles University in Prague collected samples of the natural body odors of vegetarian and meat-eating men. Women were then asked to rate the smell and attractiveness of those odors. Results showed that the odors from vegetarian men were "judged as significantly more attractive, more pleasant and less intense."

Other foods also change body odor, and not always for the better. Fatty dairy, sugar, a high-fat/low-fiber diet and even antibiotics and medication can upset the balance of good versus bad bacteria in the intestines. That, in turn, impairs the digestive process, which exacerbates body odor. Also, fried and baked goods often contain rancid fats and oils that lead to body odor. Cut back on processed foods and you will feel, look and smell sexier!

> 66 *Wear perfume wherever you want to be kissed.* 99
> —Coco Chanel

Then there is the sweat (not sweet) factor. Spicy foods make some people sweat. More sweat means more body odor. For some people, cutting out spicy foods from the diet reduces body odor. Of course, taking a daily shower and using deodorant soap wouldn't hurt, either!

Don't forget pheromones. These odor-free natural chemicals are released by glands in the skin. They float through the air and are picked up first by others' noses, then their brains (especially areas of the brain responsible for the sex drive) that ultimately end up with a reaction of either "Are you free tonight?" or "Ick. Get away from me!" All this is unconscious, since pheromones are detected at one-trillionth of a gram, so you are swept away or repulsed without a clue as to why. Pheromones are one way for the body to communicate danger, mark territory and attract a mate. High pheromone production is associated with increased frequency of sexual activity.

> **66** *Beauty is a light in the heart.* **99**
> —Kahil Gibran

There is no proof yet that food influences pheromones, but it is clear that certain foods increase libido and enhance attraction, possibly because of an as-yet-unknown pheromone response. Researchers at the Smell and Taste Research Foundation in Chicago investigated the impact of different smells on arousal in men. There was up to a 40% increase in penile blood flow when lavender and pumpkin pie were sniffed together. Other smells that enhanced libido included black licorice, orange, popcorn and vanilla.

If you want to maximize your yummy smell quotient, eat the S-Ex-Y Diet. To maximize your enjoyment, make sure you add those omega-3s, since they fine-tune the central nervous system and aid in smell acuity, so you appreciate that lavender or pumpkin aroma even more!

SCAMPROOF *your looks*

Nails: Fast-growing, hard nails are one sign of a great diet, but there is no reliable evidence that taking protein, vitamins or gelatin will strengthen nails. Even if chowing down on protein could help, gelatin is a trash protein, lacking the necessary amino acids for nail formation. Forget the rumor that calcium makes nails harder. Nails are made of protein, not calcium. However, biotin supplements (2½ milligrams/day) might help treat brittle nails, while iron-rich prunes and dark green leafies might help nails grow faster.

Hair: Despite the wealth of vitamins, fats, herbs and phytonutrients added to shampoos and conditioners, you can't nourish hair from the outside. That's because hair is dead once it grows past the scalp. All those "nutrients" are rubbed on the outside of the hair shaft and last only until the next shampoo. The only way to get rid of damaged hair is to cut it off. Don't waste your money on hair analysis, either. It doesn't detect diseases or nutritional deficiencies. There are no vitamins in hair and even though there are minerals, there is no correlation between the minerals in hair and your nutritional status. However, a bad diet will result in hair loss, dry and lifeless hair, and reduce shine. So feed your mane from the inside and keep it clean on the outside.

10 STEPS TO NOURISHING YOUR SKIN FROM WITHIN

Does your diet include all the nutrients your skin needs to stay healthy, moist, firm, glowing and young? Ask yourself the following questions to see how you're doing.

		YES	NO
1.	Do you consume 5+ servings daily of whole-grain breads and cereals? (If no, your diet may be low in the B vitamins and some trace minerals, such as chromium.)		☑
2.	Do you consume 9+ servings daily of colorful fresh fruits and vegetables, with at least 1 serving of vitamin C–rich foods (i.e., citrus fruits) and 2 servings of dark green leafy vegetables? *Hint:* Potatoes don't count, especially if they are fried. (If no, your diet could be low in vitamin C, beta-carotene, magnesium and folic acid.)		☑
3.	Do you consume at least 3 servings daily of nonfat milk or calcium-fortified soymilk or orange juice? (If no, your diet could be low in magnesium, calcium, vitamin B_2 and vitamin D.)	☑	
4.	Do you consume at least 2 servings daily of cooked dried beans and peas, extra-lean meat or chicken? (If no, your diet could be low in protein, B vitamins, iron, selenium and zinc.)		☑
5.	Do you consume at least 2 servings weekly of fatty fish, such as salmon, herring or mackerel, or several servings daily of DHA-fortified foods? (If no, your diet could be low in omega-3 fatty acids.)		☑
6.	Do you consume at least 2,000 calories daily from the foods in the S-Ex-Y Diet? (If no, consider a low-dose multiple vitamin and mineral.)		☑
7.	Do you take any medications, including birth control pills, aspirin or antacids? (These and other medications can increase the need for certain vitamins or minerals, such as B vitamins, vitamin C and iron.)		☑
8.	Do you smoke or are you around smokers? (If yes, your daily need for antioxidants and folic acid might be above average. Consume an extra citrus fruit and dark green or orange vegetable daily.)		☑
9.	Do you exercise vigorously or are you under chronic stress? (If yes, your daily requirement for vitamin C, magnesium, the trace minerals, the B vitamins and water is above average. Consume extra servings of citrus fruits, nuts, extra-lean meats and cooked dried beans and peas. Drink a minimum of 8 glasses of water daily—more if you perspire heavily.)		☑
10.	Do you live in an area with air pollution or are you outside frequently? (If yes, use sunscreen with SPF of 15 or higher. In addition, your need for the antioxidant nutrients, especially vitamins E and C, might be above average. Consider supplementing your multiple with extra vitamin E and vitamin C. Also consider using topical creams that contain antioxidants.)		☑

Feeling Great in Your Own Skin

The bottom line is that the foods that put you in the right mood, increase your energy and joie de vivre, help you maintain a stylish figure, and keep you mentally sharp are the very foods that will ageproof your appearance. Eat authentic at least 75% of the time, load the plate with antioxidant-rich foods, take the right supplements and rub some of those nutrients on the outside, and I promise that in no time you will be one of the sexiest people on the block! As one client told me after following this advice, "Once I started nourishing my looks from the inside out, I found the new me. I look great, feel great, and that energy radiates to others. When you feel good about yourself it shows, and people are naturally attracted to you. You're like a magnet. I used to be shy, but now I love to work a room!"

6

ARE YOU FIT
for sex?

THE PROMISE

Within **TWO WEEKS** of making these changes, you will

- ✓ Reduce symptoms of PMS (women only).
- ✓ Improve blood flow and circulation, thus beginning to lower the risk of a limp libido.

In **SIX MONTHS**, you will

- ✓ Increase your chances of reversing erectile dysfunction (men only).
- ✓ Increase the likelihood of being more sexually responsive, including increased sexual desire, responsiveness such as lubrication and orgasms.
- ✓ Lower the risk of all sexual-related disorders, including cancers of the breast, ovaries and prostate.
- ✓ No longer have the excuse "Not tonight, honey. I have a headache."

In **20 YEARS**, you will

- ✓ Have an increased chance of being disease-free.
- ✓ Likely be sexually active and enjoying it...a lot!

I knew from the minute I set eyes on Bob that he wasn't going to be "The One," but I can guarantee he thanks me every day for putting a spring back into his love life.

I met Bob during my four-month trial of online dating. We both knew at the first coffee date that we were a bad match, which might explain why he was so candid with me about things most men wouldn't tell their best friends. He probably figured he'd never see me again, so what did he have to lose? I heard about his recently divorced ex-wife: "I couldn't make her happy and I couldn't make her sober." I heard about his kids: "They're mad at both of us and take it out on whoever shows up." And I heard about his love life: "I'm having some real problems in the bedroom department."

Like so many men in their 50s, Bob was having trouble getting it up and keeping it up. While it was a TMI moment, I also knew I could turn this coffee date into a potentially life-changing diet consult. Super-dietitian to the rescue! I put on my diet cape and dove in with gusto.

First, I told him the obvious: "Fix your teeth, dude. No lady wants to date a guy with yellow snaggle teeth!" and "Get a new picture on your home page, because the bookcase of cinder blocks and boards in the background of your photo is a real deal breaker." Then I asked about his diet. Sure enough, what he was eating was a big-time erection blocker. I gave him the nutrition basics, with a bit of explanation thrown in, and made him raise his right hand, swearing he'd give my advice a two-month trial. When we met for our second and last coffee date, I could tell by the grin on his face that Bob was a new man!

Nine Out of Ten Could Use This Advice

Trouble in the bedroom is more common than ever. Half of men over 40 years old experience at least an occasional problem getting it up, keeping it up or ejaculating too soon, while a third say they don't even have intercourse anymore. Women's love lives are not much better, with most (almost 70%) reporting reduced desire, pain during intercourse or problems reaching orgasm. It's not that these folks are uptight or sexually suppressed. Up to 90% of reported sexual problems in both men and women do not stem from emotional issues, but are a direct result of medical disorders largely related to diet and lifestyle. That means 9 out of 10 people can turn a sluggish love life back into a whoop-dee-do affair by changing what they eat and how much they move.

> 66 *Love never dies a natural death. It dies because we don't know how to replenish its source.* 99
> —Anais Nin

Certain Circulation

It's all about circulation and circuitry. Eating authentic 75% of the time and following the guidelines of the S-Ex-Y Diet will boost your mood, sharpen your mind, eliminate fatigue and even help curb stress, all of which will translate into better boudoir behavior. The happier you are, the more likely you are to want and get sex. The more sex people report having, the happier they say they are and the younger they feel. What a great catch-22, once you jump into the cycle! Happiness and sex are great bedfellows! But you already know that. What might come as a surprise is that there also is a direct link between diet and sexual desire and performance.

The mind is the most erogenous zone, which is why sexy starts in the circuitry of the brain and works it way down. The nerve chemicals, such as dopamine, acetylcholine and norepinephrine, that help brain cells think sexy thoughts and stimulate blood flow to the sex organs depend on the foods you choose to eat. Eat junk and your nerves will be out of whack, leaving you cranky or gloomy. This explains why most people who are depressed have lost interest in sex. Eat right and nerve chemicals hum in balance, mood improves and sex drive returns. For example, nutrients such as magnesium, vitamin B_{12}, folate and tyrosine in the S-Ex-Y Diet boost dopamine and norepinephrine levels, which improves mood, mental sharpness, alertness and sex drive. But that's just the tip of the nutritional iceberg.

Feeling sexy isn't all in your head—it's also in your blood vessels. Squeaky clean, elastic arteries enable men to get it up and women to get turned on. Men need clean arteries to supply optimal blood flow to the penis for erections, and women need clean arteries for arousal. In fact, 80% of erectile dysfunction (ED) is caused by atherosclerosis. Clogged arteries shut down sex just as they shut down the heart and brain, resulting in heart disease and dementia. Anything that interferes with blood flow, from high blood pressure to obesity, dampens libido. Diabetes tops the list of causes of impotence, with hypertension and heart disease following close behind in the #2 and #3 positions, respectively. Even a cholesterol level above 239 mg/dl increases ED risk twofold.

Sexual dysfunction mirrors the epidemic of heart disease in this country. About 64 million people have heart disease and 70 million report sexual problems. The 6 million difference between those two numbers is attributed to ED and female sexual dysfunction (FSD), which precede heart disease by a few years. In fact, ED and FSD are warning signs of impending heart disease. Then there are the medications, many of which squelch sexual desire, including blood pressure meds. Sexual problems typically increase as the number of medications a person takes increases. In fact, a study from Boston University School of Medicine found that drugs prescribed to treat enlarged prostate could potentially cause irreversible sexual dysfunction in men.

Here's the clincher: Half of all men and a third of all women already have high cholesterol by their mid-20s. By the time they reach their mid-40s, half of the atherosclerotic plaque they will accumulate over their lifetimes already is firmly packed in the arteries, impeding blood flow and dampening sexual performance.

That plaque is not inevitable. It's not caused by aging. It's not necessarily a person's genetic lot in life. It's almost entirely caused by lifestyle choices. The sooner a person stops the process, the longer and more satisfying will be his or her sex life.

Mojo Maintenance

Boosting or reviving that lovin' feeling is just a heartbeat away. Literally. Follow the guidelines of the S-Ex-Y Diet and I guarantee it will give your love life a jump-start.

That's what Bob found out. He took my advice, cut back on the junk and saturated fat, loaded the plate at least 75% of the time with antioxidant-rich foods, healthy fats such as the omega-3 DHA and olive oil, whole grains, nuts and other authentic foods. He complemented that diet with a few supplements, too. As a result, his energy improved, as did his mood and ability to cope with the stresses of post-divorce life, including upset kids. He lost almost 20 pounds of blubber. His cholesterol levels dropped, as well as his blood pressure. Best of all, he was dating a woman and was hoping it would lead to some amorous evenings, which he said he was fully prepared for. Basically, Bob was a pretty happy guy.

No surprise. All aspects of sexual dysfunction improve when you fuel your body with the building blocks it needs to run like a well-tuned sex machine. You think better, feel great, sleep like a baby, handle stress better. People report that after following the S-Ex-Y Diet their love lives are more satisfying and better than ever. One study, conducted at the University of Naples, found that men following diets similar to the S-Ex-Y Diet showed improvement not only in heart-disease risk factors, but also in erectile function, while men who ate typical American diets continued to perform poorly in the bedroom. Bob definitely was feeling studlike. My clients also have confirmed that eating S-Ex-Y works. One women even told me she felt like a goddess. Feeling sexy is about the whole package—your brain, looks, fitness, energy, vitality, blood vessels and libido. The S-Ex-Y Diet takes care of it all.

Rub it on, Not into, Your Belly

A little whipped cream rubbed on a tummy or an oiled-up body might be a fun addition to a sexy romp in the hay, but it isn't pretty when that fat is packed into your belly. Oh, sure, your body needs a little fat to cushion organs and help maintain body temperature. That's taken into account when experts set ideal body weight charts. Every pound in excess of that weight is potentially messing with your love life.

A pound of body fat is about the size of a child's football. It's yellow and yucky. Now, imagine that fat tucked in and around internal organs, where it releases fats into the bloodstream, damages tissues, alters body chemistry, increases inflammation, raises levels of free radicals that pierce cell membranes and corrupts the cellular genetic code, and acts like an endocrine gland pumping out hormones that further damage organs, clog arteries, reduce sperm production and impair sexual function. Insulin and blood sugar levels rise along with risk for diabetes, while testosterone, the hormone that revs up sex drive, plummets as body fat accumulates. All that goes on 24/7, awake or asleep, watching TV or taking a shower. The longer the fat remains, the more damage to the body.

The good news? Every single one of those harmful effects are reversed or at least improved with weight loss. That's why jumping on the S-Ex-Y Weight-Loss Plan in Chapter 4 is so important. Although it's never too late to reap the rewards. With healthy and permanent weight loss, sexual desire and satisfaction improve in both men and women, symptoms of ED and FSD improve, sperm counts go up, and people say they feel younger and more vibrant, confident and full of zest. I'll take that any day over a doughnut!

ROMANTIC WAYS TO *eat the S-Ex-Y Diet*

Eating well can be sexy—just make sure to engage all the senses in the romance. Sight: Light candles or the fireplace. Sound: Add music or ocean waves. Smell: Be subtle—no cauliflower tonight! Touch: Eat with your fingers. Taste: Serve small portions that stimulate, not overwhelm (you want to leave your mouth wanting more).

1. Blindfold your lover and slowly feed him/her S-Ex-Y Diet foods, such as peeled grapes, strawberries, dark chocolate-covered almonds, watermelon cubes, whole-grain spaghetti, pomegranate seeds, slightly salted edamame beans, hunks of banana, avocado slices, fresh figs or sautéed asparagus spears.

2. Meet your lover or spouse at a bar and pretend you are meeting for the first time. Have a romantic dinner of salmon and sautéed vegetables and a glass of red wine, then go home (or to a hotel room) for your "first" romp.

3. Fill the bathtub with bubbles, light a dozen candles and feed each other bite-sized portions of your favorite healthy foods while soaking in the tub.

4. Create a romantic table for two in an unusual area of the house, such as the guest bedroom, a loft or a deck. Set the mood with candles, a pretty tablecloth, fancy dishware. Then serve two or three of your favorite dishes from the Recipe section of this book and eat with your fingers—no silverware allowed! Feed each other, too.

5. Pack an evening picnic basket filled with finger foods that are crunchy (baby carrots, nuts, apples), creamy (yogurt, peanut butter, hummus), cold (frozen blueberries), spicy (Nuts About You Curried Chicken Salad from the Recipe section) and/or sweet (fruit, Orange-Scented Swiss Kisses from the Recipe section). Add sparkling apple juice or red wine. Then watch the sunset from your favorite spot, such as the beach, on a hilltop, in a meadow or by a lake. If possible, build a campfire.

6. Skip dinner and nibble instead on S-Ex-Y foods while watching a romantic movie. Turn off the lights and light the candles or build a fire in the fireplace.

Amorous Extras

The S-Ex-Y Diet is the foundation of a lusty life. There are a few foods and supplements that also might help boost your libido, but they only work if you first follow the S-Ex-Y Diet guidelines. What are those amorous extras?

> 66 *My husband's German. Every night I get dressed up as Poland and he invades me.* 99
> —Bette Midler

While numerous herbs, from gingko to ginseng, spices including curcumin in curry powder and supplements such as tyrosine, have been studied for their ability to make you frisky, few have proven effective. However, others show definite promise. Here are the best of the best:

❶ **Arginine** This amino acid found in S-Ex-Y foods, such as nuts, seafood, watermelon, oats, green leafies and soy, is the natural equivalent of Viagra. Both increase levels of nitric oxide (NO) in the body. NO is produced in the lining (endothelium) of blood vessels. When you're sexually aroused, NO is released, which dilates blood vessels, increasing blood flow to the penis and genitalia, and resulting in an erection for a man and lubrication in a woman. In short, NO can become YES.

Supplements of arginine increase sexual desire and frequency of intercourse for both men and women, and reduce vaginal dryness in women. They also improve exercise performance and, as you'll see in Chapter 9, the more you exercise, the better sex you'll have. The optimal safe and effective dose has not been identified and may vary from one person to another. Studies have used between 500 and 2,000 milligrams/day. Arginine-rich foods also aid in weight loss, since they stimulate the production of a type of calorie-burning fat called brown adipose tissue.

❷ **Vitamin C** This vitamin helps maintain high levels of NO, possibly because it mops up free radicals that otherwise destroy NO. Vitamin C–rich foods in the S-Ex-Y Diet, such as citrus, red bell peppers, kiwi and broccoli, also enhance conversion of arginine to NO.

❸ **Soy** Limited evidence suggests that whole-soy foods, such as tofu, edamame and soymilk, help keep the vaginal area lubricated and also might help lower the risk of prostate cancer, while possibly increasing sexual desire.

4 **Yohimbine** This is the only herb approved by the U.S. Food and Drug Administration (FDA) for sexual dysfunction, especially premature ejaculation. Derived from the bark of the yohimbe tree, it increases overall blood flow to the genital area. The problem is that only pharmaceutical-grade quality has proven effective, while commercial products sold over the counter have questionable results. Take too much and yohimbine can cause anxiety and hypertension. Optimal dosage is unknown, but typical intake ranges from 15 to 30 milligrams a day, consumed in divided dosages. A combination of yohimbine and androstendione might be a better option. The latter is a building block for testosterone, the desire hormone. This combination is not advised for overweight men, since it might increase estrogen levels instead of testosterone levels. Also, it is not recommended for long-term use.

5 **Exercise** While smoking, alcohol and television viewing all have been clearly linked to a dramatic drop in sex drive, people who work out regularly and vigorously report the best sex lives, the strongest sex drives, the lustiest thoughts and the most satisfying lovemaking. Even men in their senior years who exercise daily perform in the bedroom more like their grandsons than their contemporaries. If you're bored with sex, too pooped to pucker, can't get it up or don't want to, then it's time to hit the gym or the streets before your mojo dries up and disappears! A word of caution: One study found an increase in ED in men who were enthusiastic bike riders, probably because of the compression effects of the bicycle seat. To be on the safe side, make sure to get the right fit before you take up cycling as an everyday pursuit.

Other Frisky Foils

> **"** *Give a man free hands and you'll know where to find them.* **"**
>
> —Mae West

It's hard to feel sexy if you're battling problems with the equipment. Whether it is cancer of the prostate, cervix or breast, or premenstrual syndrome (PMS), a migraine headache or a bladder infection, there is much you can do diet-wise to fix the problem and even prevent it in the first place.

The Big C

From breast and cervix to ovaries, endometrium and prostate, there is nothing funny or sexy about cancer. Many of the risk factors for cancer are outside a person's control, such as a history of infertility, failure to ovulate, a family history of cancer or living in most industrialized countries. However, more often than not, adopting the super-healthy S-Ex-Y Diet will stack the deck in favor of never having to hear the big "C" as a diagnosis at the doctor's office.

 First and foremost, keep a lean, mean figure. Excess body fat is linked to all forms of cancer, from breast to prostate.

Second, make sure you cut back on bad fats, since diets dripping in grease, including red meat, fried and fast foods, fatty dairy products and refined foods containing trans fats, are linked to inflammation and all cancers. By contrast, the healthy fats in the S-Ex-Y Diet, such as the omega-3s and olive oil, reduce inflammation, help halt abnormal cell growth associated with cancer and even enhance the effectiveness of some cancer drugs.

Third, a plate heaping with antioxidant-rich produce lowers cancer risk and helps keep the waistline slim, giving cancer a one-two punch. Make sure to include no less than nine servings a day, as is spelled out in the S-Ex-Y Diet. Include cruciferous vegetables, such as Brussels sprouts, cabbage, asparagus and kohlrabi, in the weekly menu, since they contain additional anticancer substances, called indoles. Men should include several servings daily of lycopene-rich watermelon and tomatoes to lower prostate cancer risk. Limit exposure to pesticides by choosing organic foods when possible.

Soy might be one reason why Japanese men have the lowest rate of prostate cancer and Japanese woman have the lowest risk of breast cancer in the world. Yet when they migrate to the United States and switch from tofu to steak, their risk escalates dramatically. Add a few servings of soy to your weekly diet, such as fortified soymilk or tofu. Also, include in your diet zinc-rich foods, such as oysters, whole grains, nuts, and dark green leafies to curb prostate problems.

Other compounds in the S-Ex-Y Diet, such as lignans in beans and whole grains, flavonoids in green tea and grapes, sulfuraphane in broccoli, folate in dark green leafies and polyphenols in pomegranates are directly linked to lower cancer rates in men and women. Every time you serve up a plate of S-Ex-Y, you also are protecting your body from a host of ills.

A person's best line of defense against cancer is with real food. However, a few supplements might help, too. Start with a moderate-dose multi, extra vitamin D, a calcium/magnesium supplement and the omega-3 fat DHA. Supplements of saw palmetto help combat inflammation and enlargement of the prostate in men. This herb might help regulate hormone stimulation of the prostate gland, which then reduces overstimulation. Studies have used a dosage of 160 milligrams twice daily or 320 milligrams once daily of a lipophilic extract containing 80–90% of the volatile oil. Higher amounts have proven no more effective. *(See Chapter 7.)*

Not Tonight, Honey. I Have a Headache

A headache can be brought on by the flu, eyestrain, a sinus infection, lack of sleep, a hangover, tension, cigar smoke or you name it. Even a nutrient deficiency, such as low intake of niacin, folic acid, vitamins B_1 and B_6, and pantothenic acid, can produce headaches. Large doses of vitamin B_2 improved migraine symptoms in up to 70% of women, according to one study. The S-Ex-Y Diet, rich in the omega-3s, helps prevent or treat migraine headaches, possibly by reducing spasms of blood vessels in the head and raising serotonin, the feel-good nerve chemical. Vitamin D as well as several minerals, including magnesium and calcium, are believed to aid in the management of headaches, too.

On the other hand, several substances in foods can trigger a migraine. For example,

- Tyramine, in foods, such as herring, organ meats, aged cheeses, peanuts and peanut butter; fermented sausages, such as bologna and pepperoni; chocolate; sauerkraut and alcoholic beverages.

- Tannins in apple juice, blackberries, tea and red wine. Other foods associated with headaches include milk/cheese, wheat, grapes or raisins, citrus fruits, and shellfish.

- Phenylethylamine (PEA) in chocolate affects the blood vessels and might produce migraine headaches.

- Monosodium glutamate (MSG), used as a flavor enhancer in Chinese foods and many processed foods.

- Nitrites found naturally in foods and used as preservatives in hot dogs and other processed meats.

- Coffee, wine and possibly tea are linked to headaches. Coffee withdrawal results in headaches that might linger for several days. On the other hand, 100 to 200 milligrams of caffeine can relieve regular headaches, especially when combined with painkillers like ibuprofen.

- Ice cream and icy-cold beverages can trigger migraines in some people.

Finally, keep a daily journal of your diet, exercise and sleep habits, along with any headaches that develop. After a week, review your records for patterns that might set off a headache. Develop a routine for diet, sleep and exercise, and stick with it. And avoid alcohol and tobacco.

Pee Problems

Urinary tract infections (UTI) or bladder infections are the most common kidney-related disorder in women. Symptoms include pain when urinating, frequent need to urinate, and sometimes blood in the urine. The common nutritional advice for bladder infections is to force fluids—that is, consume three to four quarts of water daily. Amp up the produce, since studies show that women who eat the most colorful produce are also at lowest risk for bladder infections. Cranberries and blueberries contain a group of phytonutrients, called tannins, that block the binding of germs to the lining of the urinary bladder, thus helping to flush these bugs out of the body and prevent or treat bladder infections. A word of warning: Check labels, since most cranberry beverages contain only 10–33% cranberry juice, and some are sweetened with highly processed pear or apple juice.

Always seek immediate medical advice for the treatment of bladder infections and always comply with medication use. To prevent bladder infections, wear cotton underwear, urinate regularly, empty the urinary bladder after intercourse, avoid bath salts or bubble bath and wipe front to back.

DE-STRESS WITH A VEGETARIAN S-Ex-Y Diet

Take the S-Ex-Y Diet one step further and go vegetarian. It might be just the ticket for lowering stress in your life. Studies, including one conducted by researchers at Arizona State University, show that people who steer clear of the steer, or any meat for that matter, have fewer negative emotions, a brighter outlook on life and lower stress scores than do meat eaters. Perhaps the added benefits come from the even higher intake of antioxidant-rich colorful produce, the phytoestrogen-rich soy, the lignan-rich whole grains, the olive oil or the vitamin- and mineral-rich diet in general. No one knows for sure, but who cares?! If you want to feel great, happy and de-stressed, then it's worth giving a vegetarian S-Ex-Y-style diet a try!

Icky Infections

There is nothing more bothersome than a yeast infection! It's caused by a bug called Candida albicans, which is a common organism found on the skin and in the mouth, digestive tract and vagina. Under normal conditions, this fungus causes no problems; the numbers are small and are kept in check by harmless bacteria. The fungus grows and symptoms develop when conditions favor their growth, such as the use of antibiotics or feminine hygiene sprays that destroy healthy bacteria. The result is vaginitis, more commonly called a yeast infection.

Lots of sugary foods or fatty junk foods in the diet encourage yeast infections, as does being diabetic or overweight. By contrast, eating the S-Ex-Y Diet with an emphasis on fish oils, nonfat plain yogurt, garlic and lots of antioxidant-rich immune-boosting produce is your best defense. *(See Chapter 7 for more on yogurt.)*

If the above dietary recommendations, combined with medication therapy, are not effective, try avoiding yeast-containing foods, such as yeasted breads, brewer's yeast and pastries made with yeast.

- Wear cotton underwear and polypropylene workout clothes.

- Use a hair dryer on a cool setting to dry the pubic area after a workout or shower.

- Sleep in cotton pajamas to allow air to circulate at night.

- Do not use feminine hygiene sprays or powders, or douche the vaginal area more than once a week.

Over-the-counter antifungal medications are now available; however, always consult a physician if you are not sure whether the condition is a yeast infection.

PMS: Pretty Miserable Sex

Premenstrual syndrome, or PMS, is the 10 days to two weeks before a woman's period when she is likely to be possessed by a cranky, depressed, anxious demon. Thoughts of romance fly out the window when she feels bloated, craves sweets instead of sex and is a bit touchy about almost anything. Up to 90% of women know what I'm talking about. All their boyfriends and husbands know, too. This is not the time to mention that she's acting like her mother or looks fat in that outfit.

Caused by hormone shifts that have a domino effect on brain chemistry and appetite, PMS can at least be curbed with the S-Ex-Y Diet. Along with balancing hormones and brain chemicals, it will help overweight women drop pounds. Since body fat acts like an endocrine gland, pumping out extra estrogen, losing weight will help lessen the hormone storm associated with PMS.

Some herbs show promise, but there is no definite proof that black cohosh, chaste berry, dong quai, St. John's wort or yarrow curb PMS symptoms. In many studies, women given these herbs or placebos report equal benefits, suggesting that just believing that a pill works is enough to improve symptoms. However, here's what does work:

- Cut out sugar and caffeine, or at least cut back, since these foods aggravate PMS. Focus instead on whole grains and starchy vegetables, such as sweet potatoes, in the S-Ex-Y Diet.

- Focus on healthy fats. Aim for at least 2 grams a day of the omega-3s, EPA and DHA, during the PMS phase, by increasing your intake of seafood or foods fortified with an algal-based DHA. Also, consider supplementing during this time with 3 grams a day of evening primrose oil.

- Eat the Ménage à Trois breakfast, have a Quickie snack midmorning, a Twosome lunch and a G-Spot snack midafternoon. Little meals and snacks of real food throughout the day curb cravings and keep brain chemistry balanced.

- Add soy. Estrogenlike compounds, called phytoestrogens or isoflavones, in soy foods help curb the body's natural hormone swells, reducing mood swings, hot flashes and other PMS symptoms. Stick to real food, not supplements, to get the right balance of isoflavones.

- Load up on magnesium-rich foods in the S-Ex-Y Diet, such as whole grains, wheat germ, nuts, legumes and dark green leafies. Magnesium levels drop during PMS, which contributes to water retention, cramping, headaches, stress and an oversensitive nervous system.

- Focus on calcium. Mood and concentration problems subside when women consume at least 1,300 milligrams of calcium-rich foods in their daily diets, such as nonfat milk or yogurt, calcium-fortified soymilk or orange juice and canned salmon with the bones.

- Take a moderate-dose multivitamin and mineral, plus extra vitamin D (about 1,000 IU a day). Also, consider taking a vitamin B$_6$ supplement

(50–150 milligrams/day) starting on day 10 of the menstrual cycle and continuing through day 3 of the next cycle.

- Limit salt to reduce bloating.

- Exercise! Women who are in great physical shape are least likely to suffer from PMS symptoms.

Men—Yes! Pause—No!

Hormones go haywire during and after menopause. Testosterone and estrogen both decline during menopause. Lower testosterone produces a limp libido and reduced estrogen dries up the vagina, making sex uncomfortable or even painful. Many medications to treat heart disease, such as beta-blockers and diuretics, only worsen the problem with side effects including problems with arousal. Depression accompanying menopause lowers sex drive, while most drugs used to treat depression also cause performance and libido problems. Wow. This sounds like living hell! But wait. There is much you can do to side step the side effects of menopause and even avoid having to take medication.

Hormone replacement therapy (HRT) that includes both estrogen and progesterone (and possibly a touch of testosterone) is the first line of defense, at least from a medical standpoint. Or, if you are opposed to pills, try a topical estrogen cream or estrogen ring, which is placed in the vagina and slowly releases estrogen locally. Over the counter lubricating gels also replenish vaginal moisture.

Then there is diet and exercise. Maintaining a desirable body weight by following the S-Ex-Y Diet and exercise plan helps curb menopausal symptoms, from hot flashes to depression. Women who are at a healthy weight and who eat well also suffer the least during the menopausal years and are less likely to need HRT. Daily exercise also balances hormones and revs sex drive. Consider it a must-do to navigate the menopausal years.

Soy is worth a try. Estrogen-like compounds, called phytoestrogens, found in soybeans can help offset the drop in a woman's natural estrogen. While not exactly like estrogen, phytoestrogens act much like the female hormone, binding to the body's estrogen receptors and supplementing the effects of estrogen when levels are low. How much is enough? Preliminary evidence suggests that as little as 15 ounces of soymilk or 2 ounces of tofu daily might be all a woman needs to help dampen the hot flash and curb the estrogen swells during menopause.

Other tricks that might ease the symptoms include:

- Avoiding coffee, chocolate, alcohol and spicy foods, all of which alter blood flow and can increase the symptoms of hot flashes.

- Eating small meals and snacks regularly throughout the day. Large meals increase body temperature and might aggravate a hot flash.

- Placing a glass of ice water by the bed at night to drink at the first sign of an approaching night sweat. Try opening the bedroom window to keep the cool air flowing, using 100% cotton sheets and a small fan by the bed.

- Being careful about herb teas. Some herbs, such as black cohosh or dong quai, cause blood vessel dilation and could aggravate a hot flash.

- Dressing in layers, so you can add or subtract clothes as your body's temperature fluctuates.

Strut Your Stuff

> 66 *From the moment I was six I felt sexy. And let me tell you it was hell, sheer hell, waiting to do something about it.* 99
> —Bette Davis

Feeling sexy, confident and passionate about life is far too important for a vibrant life to settle for less. Even if you don't feel in the mood at first, dive into the romance game anyway. Don't wait to be "in the mood." Act as if you feel sexy. Fake it until you make it. Jumping back into romance (with the right attitude, of course!) is enough to rekindle the flames. Going through the motions often is all it takes to generate the feelings. One study found that women given placebos to treat a low libido reported improvements in their sex lives, desires, arousal, number and strength of orgasms and enjoyment of the whole experience.

Instead of getting into bed thinking, "Oh, here we go again. This will never work," adopt a "Let's go for it" attitude. Hope for good things, then make them happen. Strut your stuff, baby!

7

DO YOU EMBRACE

mother nature's aphrodisiacs?

THE PROMISE

Within **TWO WEEKS** of making these changes, you will

- ✓ Have more energy, so you'll be more inter-ested in and motivated for romance.
- ✓ Begin to appreciate the flavor of foods, other than just salt.
- ✓ Begin to wonder why you ever liked libido-lowering junk food.

In **SIX MONTHS**, you will

- ✓ Think more clearly.
- ✓ Feel less stressed.
- ✓ Have reduced inflam-mation, thus lowering risk for disease and sexual problems.
- ✓ Have improved hor-mone balance.
- ✓ Notice an improvement in mood.

In **20 YEARS**, you will

- ✓ Have slowed brain aging.
- ✓ Feel great and sexier.

The notion that certain foods have a wake-up-and-smell-the-coffee effect on your love life is older than the Kama Sutra. Long before Adam met Eve, Cleopatra met Mark Antony, or Casanova romanced all of Venice, food was intimately linked to love. We often speak of "eating our hearts out," "feasting our eyes" or having "lusty appetites." We call our lovers "spicy," "a dish," "a hot tomato" or "'good enough to eat." It is a very thin line separating sexual appetite and physical hunger.

Aphrodisiacs—named after Aphrodite, the Greek goddess of sexual rapture and the mother of Cupid—have graced menus before there were tables. The moon and almost everything underneath it have been touted as aphrodisiacs. Most are useless; all are interesting. There is a method to this madness, with unspoken folklore fueling what might be and what definitely doesn't have aphrodisiac potential. To qualify, a food must meet at least one of the following criteria:

1 **It looks sexy.** Some of the first aphrodisiacs developed their reputation based on shape, a belief called the Doctrine of Signatures. This belief—the ultimate food porn—holds that the universe reveals the use or virtues of a food by its appearance. For example, ginseng root is famous as an aphrodisiac because it has leglike appendages and resembles the human body (the term *ginseng* means "man root"). The rare root that sprouts an extra appendage resembling the sexual organ sells for thousands of dollars in some countries. Other organ lookalikes have included bananas, asparagus, carrots, oysters, avocados (fruits of what the Aztecs called the "testicle tree") and figs.

2 **It smells sexy.** Foods that stimulate the senses are considered pleasurable, hence sexy. Foods that are creamy, smooth, rich or spicy, such as chocolate (perhaps laced with a little chili powder), have made it on the Love Potions #9 list.

3 **It acts sexy.** Fertile animals have graced the tables of many candlelit dinners, if only because there is hope their revved-up fertility will be passed along to the diner. Fertilized eggs have been slurped by many a lover, while rabbits gained notoriety in some areas of the world for this reason.

4 **It is housed with sexy.** Seafood that comes from the land of Aphrodite—who was said to have risen from sea foam where Uranus's genitals fell in battle—has at one time or another adopted a sexy aura. Hence, clams, lobsters, fish eggs, eels and sea slugs once had racy reputations.

5 **It reminds us of sexy.** Foods filled with seeds, such as pomegranates and figs, are linked with enhanced sexual desire, for obvious reasons.

6 **It makes us feel sexy.** Foods, such as chili, curried dishes and other spicy foods, that increase body temperature have been thought to arouse passion.

The most ridiculous reason of all for a food to grace the aphrodisiac list is that it is rare or new. This questionable quality explains why white bread and potatoes at one time were considered passion foods and why people once snacked on dried salamander and fat of camel's hump. Ick!

LUSTY *tidbits*

1. Have you used the term *horny* to describe being sexually aroused? It is likely this term comes from Asian countries where there was a widespread belief that ground-up horns of various animals, such as rhinoceros and reindeer, could be powerful aphrodisiacs (probably because of their phallic shape). Some people went so far as to recommend unicorn horn; but finding a supplier was darn near impossible.

2. The ancient Greeks spread barley around the temple of Demeter to symbolize semen ejaculation and to ensure fertility. The custom was passed down through the ages, and today we throw rice at the bride and groom during weddings.

3. In jolly ol' England, to woo a lover, one mixed flour, water and lard, sprinkled the dough with saliva, then placed it between the legs to give it the form and scent of the spell caster. The loaf was baked and offered to the object of desire.

You may laugh, or gag, at some of these beliefs, but modern-day aphrodisiacs are no better. Nutrient cocktails made from herbs, vitamins and extracts are billed as climax-enhancers, when typically all they contain is caffeine or niacin, substances that produce a temporary flushing of the skin, mistaken for arousal. Anything with hormonelike compounds, from truffles (that contain the male pig hormone, androstenol, and also are called "testicles of the earth") or flaxseed (which contains a natural hormonelike compound called lignin), are touted as love potions. Unfortunately, these compounds have little or no sexual-enhancing effect on humans when eaten in food. Even the foods associated with good times and pleasure, and that people typically say make them crave sex, such as pasta, ice cream, champagne and whipped cream, have no basis in scientific fact, which is why the U.S. Food and Drug Administration (FDA) reports that all products and foods sold over the counter as aphrodisiacs are hogwash.

Of course, if you believe something is going to work, then it probably will. A study from the University of Michigan found that giving people a pretend pill and telling them it enhanced pleasure was enough to trigger the brain to produce its own opioids to ease pain. If we can be tricked into making our own natural painkiller, why not our own natural love potions? Believing that a certain food induces desire is enough to be a self-fulfilling prophecy. In the realm of folklore, imagination is not to be ignored. And, in the end, what does it matter? If it works, it works!

Help! I Need an Aphrodisiac

Cupid doesn't always use an arrow—sometimes he uses a fork. There are a few foods, when added to the S-Ex-Y Diet, that can help you get "in the mood," while sharpening your mind and reducing stress. Combine what you have learned throughout this book about authentic foods and when to eat them with the super-sexy foods in this chapter and you are guaranteed to feel amazing, improve your self-confidence, feel sexier in your skin and even drop a few pounds. In short, feed the soul, feed the body and you feed your sexy self.

Let me emphasize that the real aphrodisiacs are the ones you eat for breakfast, lunch and dinner, day after day on the S-Ex-Y Diet. All foods in this plan get as much nutrition from as few calories as possible. To qualify as a super-sexy food, it must take that message to the next level. These foods not only are packed with nutrition, they also meet at least two of the following criteria. They

1. Balance hormones.
2. Enhance metabolism.
3. Improve blood flow, by keeping blood vessels clean and/or raising nitric oxide levels.
4. Boost mood.
5. Reduce inflammation.
6. Protect brain and skin cells from damage and aging.

There are lots of great foods that fulfill this criteria. In fact, mixing and matching a variety of authentic foods is the key to getting the best protection against disease and aging, while maximizing your efforts to feel, look and think great—the magic combo for sexy. I could write a book the size of Wikipedia on super-sexy foods alone. But I have only one chapter, so I've chosen my favorite dozen. All are easy to find, supported by an ocean of research on their health-enhancing benefits and are within most people's food budget. (I am not an advocate of the latest—and expensive—designer fruit or fad juice, in case you haven't noticed!)

Never fear—you don't have to cook up a storm of bizarre foods to get to first base. In many cases, you don't even need to know how to cook to include these tasty treats in your diet. (BTW: If you come across a food you think should be included in this list and want to know my opinion of it, send me a message on my website [www.elizabethsomer.com]. I'll give you my "yeah" or "nay.")

HONORABLE
amorous mentions

Avocados	Oranges	Oysters	Chewy whole grains
Nuts	Tomatoes	Garnet sweet potatoes	Red bell peppers
Dried plums	Olive oil	Winter squash	Mushrooms

Amorous Edibles: The Naughty Dozen

Do these aphrodisiacs really work? Friends, clients and I have given all of them the "sex test," including them along with the S-Ex-Y Diet for a trial run of at least six months. Results? Yahoo! Here are just a few comments at the end of the test (the names have been changed to protect the reputations of the not-so-innocent. Many of these people are parents and some are grandparents, so their children and grandkids definitely don't want to know some of this stuff!).

- *Debbie:* "We had a great sex life but, hey, I was willing to try an aphrodisiac or two. No matter how good it is, it always can be better, right? And it was!"

- *Steven:* "I'm still not sure whether it was the salmon or the candles, but my wife and I both agree that a few weeks of these foods sure amped up our love life!"

- *Wendy:* "After watching the movie *9½ Weeks,* we tried the scene where the actor blindfolds the actress and feeds her aphrodisiacs, like strawberries and watermelon. Wow. What a turn-on!"

Add the following dozen as often as possible to your weekly S-Ex-Y Diet and I promise you will be thanking me big time in no time!

1. Salmon

Salmon is the ultimate aphrodisiac. It is high in protein, B vitamins, potassium to keep the heart pumping in rhythm and astaxanthin, and a potent antioxidant. The omega-3s in fatty fish, especially docosahexaenoic acid (DHA), improve mood, sharpen the mind, keep blood vessels squeaky clean and reduce inflammation. They lower heart disease risk; raise HDLs—the good cholesterol—help stabilize the heartbeat; reduce blood clots, thereby curbing the risk for heart attack and stroke; and lower the chances of getting high blood pressure, cancer, vision loss, arthritis, depression, attention deficit, dementia and a host of other unsexy ills. These omega-3s even improve fertility in men.

How much? Include at least two 4-ounce servings weekly, or take a supplement. Choose wild salmon when it is affordable, since it is higher in omega-3s and vitamin D and lower in contaminants, such as PCBs and pesticides found in farmed salmon. (If the package says *Atlantic salmon*, it's farmed.) Canned salmon is good, too.

Eat more. Grill, bake, broil or poach. Make a sandwich spread with canned salmon, fat-free mayonnaise, diced celery and herbs. Have lox and bagels (use fat-free cream cheese). Try the Bedded Herbed Salmon in the Recipe section.

2. Dark Greens

These are some of the most mood- and energy-enhancing foods on the planet. Calorie for calorie, you get more vitamins, minerals, phytonutrients and fiber than almost any other food. Greens clean arteries, protect brain cells from aging and depression, and improve blood flow to all body parts, thus lowering the risk for heart disease, cancer, vision loss, stroke, dementia, high blood pressure, wrinkling and skin cancer, erectile dysfunction, and loss of libido. They are rich in antioxidants, potassium, B vitamins, vitamin C, magnesium, calcium, zinc, iron, chlorophyll and a host of phytonutrients from carotenoids to polyphenols and betaine. You honestly can't get to sexy without them!

How much? At least two servings a day of the darkest greens you can find. A serving is 1 cup raw or ½ cup cooked.

Eat more. Include a spinach or baby greens salad at lunch, such as the Zesty Shrimp and Spinach Salad in the Recipe section. Mix greens into other foods, such as mashed potatoes, soups or stews. Layer into sandwiches. Sauté chard, kale, mustard, collard or beet greens in olive oil and garlic.

> **"** *A half cup of blueberries has the antioxidants of five apples.* **"**

3. Berries

In France, strawberries are considered an aphrodisiac and are served at weddings. The antioxidant mix in berries is so powerful that they rank right along with salmon and greens as the most nutritious foods in the diet. A half cup of blueberries has the antioxidants of five apples. Phytonutrients, such as anthocyanins, resveratrol, ellagic acid, carotenoids and polyphenols, protect healthy cells throughout the body, preventing aging from head to groin. They lower risk for heart disease, cancer, diabetes, vision loss, urinary tract infections, inflammation, erectile dysfunction, periodontal disease and kidney stones. Ellagic acid in berries is a youth elixir for skin, increasing elastin fibers and inhibiting collagenase, an enzyme that otherwise breaks down collagen in the skin. Berries' ability to protect your mind is so amazing that some call them "brain berries." They also are rich in fiber, folate, vitamin C and potassium.

How much? One cup a day, most days of the week. The antioxidant power is directly proportional to the color, so select the darkest berries that are richly hued from skin to core. Choose fresh or plain frozen (make sure there is no sugar added), wild berries, when possible, and preferably organic, since berries are on the Dirty Dozen list when it comes to pesticides. No quick fix here. You can't get any of the benefits of berries in a pill. In fact, one study found that of hundreds of berry supplements studied, about half had no active ingredients at all. On the other hand, black rice bran also is high in one of the antioxidants found in berries—anthocyanins. Add it to dishes on occasion as a substitute.

Eat more. Eat berries plain, or use them in sauces, salads, smoothies, desserts such as Berry Quickie Ice Cream Pie in the Recipe section, muffins, tarts and as toppings.

THE DIRTY dozen

Should you buy organic produce? It depends. Some conventionally grown produce is almost pesticide-free, according to the Environmental Working Group, a nonprofit organization that protects the public. No need to go organic when it comes to onions, avocados, corn, pineapple, mangoes, sweet peas, asparagus, kiwi, canned peaches, blueberries, cabbage, eggplant, cantaloupe, watermelon, grapefruit or sweet potatoes. But you might want to spend the extra cash for organic when purchasing these fruits and vegetables:

1. Celery	4. Raspberries	7. Bell peppers	10. Cherries
2. Fresh peaches	5. Apples	8. Spinach	11. Imported grapes
3. Strawberries	6. Nectarines	9. Kale	12. Pears

Even organic produce may contain pesticides, but at one-third the level of conventional. To further reduce the risk of ingesting toxins from pesticides, wash and scrub, then peel and discard outer leaves. Eat a variety of different produce for a better mix and to reduce pesticide exposure from any one fruit or vegetable. A few studies show that organic produce is higher in phytonutrients, antioxidants and vitamin C. However, keep in mind that the benefits of eating colorful conventional produce *far* outweigh any tiny, potential risk of pesticides or slight reduction in nutrients, and especially when compared to not eating produce at all.

4. Pomegranates

There is something super-sexy about clusters of densely packed, ruby-red kernels bursting with juice. No wonder the 800+ garnet-colored jeweled seeds inside this fruit have long been the symbol of longevity, immortality and abundance in China, and fertility in Greece. Called the "love apple," some suspect it was a pomegranate, not an apple, that tempted Adam and Eve in the Garden of Eden, while legend has it that humans become immortal by eating these seeds.

Pomegranates are not likely to turn a couch potato into Casanova, but they are rich in potassium, vitamin C, fiber, B vitamins and phytonutrients like polyphenols, anthocyanins and procyanidins. (A cup of pomegranate juice has more than 10 times the polyphenols of apple juice, 639 versus 61 milligrams!) They have three times the antioxidants of green tea, and help lower the risk for inflammation, heart disease, dementia and Alzheimer's, cancer, male infertility, high blood pressure and damage to the genetic code; improve blood flow to all parts of the body, including the genitals; and even help reverse atherosclerosis, the underlying cause of heart disease and erectile dysfunction. A phytonutrient, called punicalagin, speeds healing and builds collagen and elastin that plump and firm the skin.

How much? Sprinkle a tablespoon or more of pomegranate seeds into foods at least four times a week from fall through winter when these fruits are available, or use pure pomegranate juice throughout the year. Packaged seeds (POM Wonderful Arils) are available in the refrigerated section of select stores from October through January.

Eat more. Sprinkle seeds into salads, desserts and fruit, rice and pasta dishes. Add juice to sauces, dressings and marinades. Try the Fall Romance Salad in the Recipe section. To seed, put in a bowl of water, peel away the white and allow seeds to sink, which makes separating the pith from the fruit easier.

an apple today, OR YESTERDAY?

The claim that fruits and vegetables are less nutritious today than in the past is unfounded, according to comparisons of past and present data by the U.S. Department of Agriculture (USDA). There also is no credible evidence to support the claim that farming has depleted the soil. In fact, this goes against what experts know about plant growth. For example, spinach needs iron. If that mineral was depleted from the soil, spinach leaves would be pale and small. Plants make their own vitamins and fiber, so soil quality has little to do with determining levels of these.

5. Whole Soy Foods

Whole soy foods are rich in protein, iron, calcium, magnesium, B vitamins, antioxidants and a host of phytonutrients, such as saponins, phytosterols, phenolic compounds, phytic acid and protease inhibitors. However, they are best known for their phytoestrogens, weak hormonelike compounds that help balance estrogen levels in a woman's body, possibly reducing hot flashes and premenstrual mood swings, stabilizing blood sugar, and even aiding in arousal. Soy also lowers risk for heart disease, hormone-related cancers, diabetes, high blood pressure, dementia, wrinkling, inflammation, skin cancer and bone loss, while increasing nitric oxide, which improves blood flow to the sex organs.

How much? Up to 3 servings a day for people with no history of breast cancer. Limit to one a day otherwise. Don't take shortcuts by using processed soy products and supplements, since it is the mix of compounds in whole soy foods that act synergistically to lower disease risk and promote health.

Eat more. Substitute tofu for meat in casseroles, soups and stews. Use cooked soybeans instead of garbanzos in hummus. Add edamame to stir-frys. Use soymilk instead of milk in recipes.

6. Watermelon

What better way to improve health—physically, mentally and sexually—than to nibble on sweet and juicy, chin-dribbling watermelon?! Watermelon is an excellent source of lycopene, a red pigment that lowers heart disease and heart-attack risk. In fact, watermelon has more lycopene than tomatoes do—up to 20 milligrams in each 2-cup serving. The lycopene in watermelon helps lower risk for inflammation, prostate cancer, urinary tract infections, skin damage, vision and bone loss, and possibly even weight gain. Watermelon also is low or free of cholesterol, fat and sodium, and is a good source of arginine and citrulline, amino acids that maintain the blood vessels, increase nitric oxide and improve blood flow to all tissues. Vitamins A and C in watermelon show promise in lowering risk for cancers of the esophagus, stomach, lungs, liver, cervix, colon and pancreas. This fruit is a natural hydrator, containing 92% water, and a great source of potassium, magnesium, the antioxidant glutathione and vitamin B_6. The seeds are a rich source of protein, magnesium, iron and zinc.

How much? You need approximately 10 milligrams of lycopene a day from a variety of sources (including tomato products, guava and pink grapefruit), or the equivalent of 1 cup of watermelon daily. Watermelon stored and served at room temperature is higher in lycopene and vitamins than chilled watermelon.

Eat more. Carry bags of sliced or cubed watermelon for an on-the-go snack. Toss in salads, salsas and smoothies. Top yogurt with watermelon cubes. Blend watermelon and Splenda and freeze for a homemade sorbet. Purée watermelon, sweeten with concentrated apple juice, freeze into ice cubes or pops, then add cubes to club soda for a refreshing drink.

7. Wheat Germ

The heart of the wheat kernel is a gold mine of nutrition. A ½-cup serving of toasted wheat germ supplies more than half of a person's daily magnesium needs, a mineral that three out of four people don't get enough of, yet is essential for reducing stress, building bones and regulating thyroid function and heart rate. People cut their risk of developing diabetes by 48% when they consume magnesium-rich diets. Wheat germ also supplies healthy amounts of vitamins, including folic acid, vitamin E, iron and zinc, as well as hefty doses of phytonutrients, such as phytosterols that reduce cholesterol absorption and lower heart disease risk, octacosanol that increases muscle stamina, and ergothionine, a potent antioxidant.

How much? Just 2 tablespoons a day supply 4 grams of protein, 2 grams of fiber, a third of your vitamin E needs and a big dose of other nutrients.

Eat more. Sprinkle on oatmeal or yogurt, add to cookie and pancake batters, mix into muffin or meat loaf recipes, or blend with honey and peanut butter for a sandwich spread.

8. Figs

First cultivated in Egypt, figs made their way through Crete, Greece and on to Rome, where they were considered a sacred fruit. The Dutch painters in the 17th and 18th centuries used figs as a symbol of sexuality and fertility. The seeds are the real fruit, since the fig is actually a flower inverted into itself. Fresh or dried, Black Mission, Kadota, Calimyrna or Adriatic, figs are rich in both soluble and insoluble fiber, which improves blood flow and helps balance blood sugar levels. The soluble pectin in figs lowers cholesterol nearly as well as some medications. Figs are good sources of vitamins A, E and the Bs, as well as magnesium, potassium, calcium, iron and manganese. Only fresh figs are high in vitamin C. Their claim to fame is their high antioxidant content, and their special mix of amino acids, believed to increase libido and sexual stamina.

How much? Aim for four servings a week. A serving is ½ cup raw or ¼ cup dried. Some dried fruits are processed with sulfites to preserve color. Choose sulfite-free, organic figs if you are sensitive to these additives.

Eat more. Stuff figs with low-fat cheeses and nuts for a snack or appetizer, add them to fat-free cottage cheese or oatmeal (as in the Sensuous Honeyed

Fig Oatmeal in the Recipe section), poach them in red wine and serve them with yogurt. Add to rice dishes, desserts, batters, smoothies and salads. Purée and use them as a replacement for fat in baking. Even eating a fresh fig is a sensual experience: Make two cross slits halfway through, then gently press to turn the fig inside out so the pulpy flesh is exposed. Suck each petal of skin to remove the flesh.

9. Yogurt

A Greek custom for newlyweds is to eat yogurt with honey and nuts before their honeymoon to ensure prosperity and fertility. Yogurt is a rich source of mood- and mind-boosting nutrients, including protein, calcium, B vitamins, magnesium, potassium and zinc. Yogurt that contains Lactobacillus acidophilus, Bifidobacterium and L. rhamnosus (called probiotics) improves immune function and reduces the risk for certain allergies, intestinal problems, ulcers, cancer, urinary tract infections and yeast infections in women. The healthy bacteria in yogurt promotes vaginal health, lowers blood pressure and also helps lower cholesterol levels, thus reducing heart-disease risk.

The combination of protein and calcium in yogurt might aid in weight loss. Researchers at the University of Tennessee found that obese adults who ate three servings daily of fat-free yogurt lost 22% more weight and 61% more fat than those who ate the same calories without the yogurt.

> **How much?** One cup a day to supply a daily dose of up to 10 billion organisms, preferably a variety of strains rather than a single strain. The National Yogurt Association has a "live active cultures" (LAC) seal guaranteeing that a yogurt contains at least 100 million bacteria per gram at the time of manufacture. (Use before the expiration date on the label, since the bacteria count drops dramatically after that.) Probiotics do not permanently adhere to the intestinal lining, but exert their benefits as they metabolize and move through the intestines, so consume yogurt daily.

> **Eat more.** Skip the fruited and flavored yogurts, which have the sugar equivalent of a candy bar. Instead, sweeten plain regular, goat or Greek yogurt with a bit of jam, fresh fruit or honey at home. Include yogurt in snacks, dips, toppings, or salad dressings as a replacement for sour cream, or in chilled soups, desserts or parfaits. Plain, unsweetened kefir is good, too.

10. Fresh Herbs and Spices

Both fresh and dried herbs and spices stimulate the senses and enhance the sensuality of any dish. They also are gold mines of antioxidants and anti-inflammatory compounds that improve memory and blood flow, lower disease risk, and enhance sexual performance and desire. They contain anti–blood clotting and antimicrobial compounds. Ginger stimulates the senses, eases muscle pain, soothes nausea and thins the blood. Nutmeg and cloves increase sexual desire (at least in animals), black pepper and cayenne boost metabolism, basil has been used for centuries to heighten sex drive, chili pepper and curry rev circulation, curcumin protects the brain from dementia, rosemary eliminates cancer-causing substances formed during the cooking of meat, and oregano is rich in the antioxidant phytonutrients limonene, linalol, and thymol that protect skin from aging and damage. Saffron, which improves sexual function and alleviates erectile dysfunction, contains picrocrocin, a chemical that heightens the body's sensitivity to touch. Spearmint, peppermint, dill and sage are rich in phenolic compounds that reduce inflammation. Cinnamon helps normalize blood sugar. Adding chili powder and capsaicin to the daily diet has a slight metabolism-boosting effect that equates to about 50 extra calories a day, which means up to a 5-pound loss of body weight in one year, according to a study conducted by researchers at Pennington Biomedical Research Center in Baton Rouge. Vanilla comes from the Spanish word for vagina, since its flavor and aroma are both calming and sexually arousing. In a study from the Smell and Taste Treatment and Research Foundation in Chicago, men who smelled vanilla had a 40% increased blood flow to the genitals.

> **How much?** At least 1 teaspoon daily dried or 1 tablespoon daily fresh. Vary herbs and spices from day to day. Choose fresh over dried when possible, since fresh herbs and spices contain more antioxidants.

> **Eat more.** Use instead of salt to season and flavor all recipes.

11. Dark Chocolate

Believe it or not, chocolate started out as a medicine, not a vice. Thanks once again to the Greeks, chocolate was soon catapulted to heavenly status when it was named Theobroma, or "Food of the Gods." It was used by the Aztecs to treat hundreds of ailments. Chocolate is one of Mother Nature's best sources of polyphenols, which are antioxidants, anti-inflammatories, anticancer, antiviral and antifungal. Polyphenols in cocoa powder protect cholesterol from

> **" Women who eat dark chocolate report more satisfying sex lives. "**

oxidation by free radicals, so they are less likely to stick to arteries and most likely to decrease the risk for atherosclerosis, dementia and erectile dysfunction. They protect the genetic code within each cell, lower skin cancer and wrinkling, and reduce dementia risk.

Compounds in chocolate lower blood pressure and strengthen blood vessels, all of which make for great lovemaking. In fact, women who eat dark chocolate report more satisfying sex lives. Caffeine, arginine, phenylethylamines (PEA), and a host of nutrients, from B vitamins to magnesium and iron, all stimulate brain chemistry to improve mood, calm the body, trigger sexual desire, boost nitric oxide levels and even give you that tickle in the middle that reminds you of being in love. Anandamides (meaning "bliss" in Sanskrit) target cannabinoid receptors in the brain, much like marijuana, to give a pleasurable high. And chocolate releases morphinelike compounds in the brain, called endorphins, that produce lusty, pleasurable feelings.

How much? No more than 1 ounce a day of dark chocolate with at least 70% cocoa powder. Avoid Dutch processed cocoa, since alkaline compounds destroy the polyphenols.

Eat more. Who needs suggestions on how to eat chocolate!? Are you kidding me? Eat it any way you like; drink it any way you love; or rub, sprinkle and pour it on your lover and lick it off!

12. Red Wine

Wine is the universal love potion. It increases sexual desire and responsiveness in both men and women, and aids in lubrication for women, probably because it suppresses any fear or guilt about improper behavior, allowing the imbiber to "loosen up." A study from Spain found that resveratrol in red wine also aids in weight loss, enhancing fat burning and reducing cells' ability to make and store fat. Of course, get too friendly with the bottle and your mojo will morph into a parked car. As Shakespeare so succinctly wrote in Macbeth: "It [alcohol] provides the desire, but it takes away the performance."

How much? One 5-ounce glass of red wine a day for women and no more than two glasses for men. Sip, don't gulp, since resveratrol is absorbed 100-fold better through the mucus membranes in the mouth than it is from the intestines.

Eat more. Drink with a meal, rather than before, to help curb excess intake.

HIGH-RANKING unsexy foods

Any food with more calories than nutrients eaten in excess is a super de-sexer. A diet with humongous portions, too much processed foods and sugar, and too little produce and omega-3s is a wish list for feeling frumpy and dumpy. Here are the worst offenders:

1. Meat and full-fat dairy Red meat not only sours body odor *(see Chapter 5)*, plugs your arteries, and increases risk for memory loss, it also increases the risk for erectile dysfunction and dampens a man's performance in the bedroom. Researchers at the University of Utah School of Medicine report that blood testosterone levels plunged 50% in a group of men after a high-fat meal.

2. Refined grains People who eat refined grains are the most likely to be overweight. Packing excess body weight also leads to performance problems. Unfit and fat men are much more likely to battle erectile dysfunction, compared to men who stay fit and lean in their second 50 years. Overweight women are most likely to not feel sexy or have trouble with arousal. These foods even may lead to hearing loss, which means you won't know when that special someone is asking for your number!

3. Commercial snack foods Chips, cookies, crackers, pretzels, candy, cheese puffs, energy or granola-like bars, cinnamon rolls, muffins, pork rinds, buttered popcorn…the list is endless when it comes to highly processed, overly salted and sugared, greasy junk that comes in a bag, box, carton or container. Every bite you take leads you one step away from your sexy self.

4. Plastic bottles A chemical found in plastic water bottles and metal cans, called bisphenol A or BPA, acts as a weak estrogen, which can upset hormones and even increase the risk for cancer. Instead, choose fresh or frozen foods instead of canned. Purchase acidic foods, such as tomatoes, in glass containers. Wash hands after handling receipts. Sip from steel or glass containers and avoid plastics with the "code 7" on the bottom.

5. Bagged popcorn Chemicals, called perfluorooctanioic acid or PFOAs, in the lining of the bag are suspected to cause infertility, according to a UCLA study. In animals, PFOAs also cause testicular and pancreatic cancers. Microwaving causes the chemicals to vaporize and saturate the popcorn.

Sexy is as Much about the Mood as the Food

Romance has a lot more to do with "chemistry," lingering glances and subtle body language than it does with aphrodisiacs. It has more to do with what's between the ears than what's going on between the legs. Besides, most of us are not likely to choose lovers who are so uptight about sex that they force themselves to eat goat's testicles for breakfast or sprinkle rhino horn on their pasta in the midst of a candlelit dinner.

The delicious complexities that attract you to someone are likely to include qualities such as humor, intelligence, vulnerability and integrity, not sexual prowess alone. Good old common sense, combined with presentation when it comes to food, will go a lot further than the most potent "love potion" in boosting energy and health. All you need is the S-Ex-Y Diet, laced with the Dozen Amorous Edibles, along with a bit of fitness thrown in and you have the magic potion for feeling even more amorous and sexy.

There are lots of foods that can make a perfectly respectable woman (or man) feel like a floozy (or stud). In fact, almost any food can be sexy if eaten with abandon. That little romantic meal is all about setting the mood, then giving in to healthy temptation. Subtle is sexier than "in your face." You want a whisper, not a shout. Here are just a few ideas that are simple, elegant (or slightly risqué) and guaranteed to perk up your love life.

- Feed each other watermelon chunks and dark chocolate bits on the floor in front of a fire.

- Picnic in the backyard on a fuzzy blanket and feast on champagne, strawberries and frozen blueberries.

- Steam mussels in wine and herbs, serve with chunks of sourdough French bread, and let the juice dribble down your chin.

- Feed each other Rum-ba Crumble Love* blindfolded.

- Peel grapes and feed them to your lover one by one.

- Pack a picnic lunch that includes juicy fruits, such as mangos, papaya, oranges and honeydew melon. Eat the fruit with your fingers.

- Rent a copy of your favorite sexy movie *(see Chapter 1 for suggestions)*. Take notes, then plan your own food orgy.

- Serve your lover breakfast in bed, including fresh-squeezed orange juice and an Apple-of-My-Eye Popover Pancake* with fresh raspberries.

- Drive out to the country. Pick wildflowers by the side of the road, then picnic in a vacant field, hopefully one with a view.

- Stop at the local seafood market at the beach, buy a whole cooked crab and a bottle of sparkling apple juice or champagne. Sit on the cliff above the ocean, eat cracked crab and toast to your love.

- Have a giggle-fest. Toss nuts, grapes, berries or air-popped popcorn into the air and catch the bits in your mouth. Have a cherry–pit spitting contest.

- Eat sushi, chocolate pudding, baby carrots dunked in spicy hummus or any super-flavorful or creamy textured food with your eyes closed, savoring the taste, texture and smell.

- Kidnap your lover. Drive him/her around town until totally lost, then pull up to a favorite restaurant for a candlelit dinner.

- Eat spaghetti, sorbet with fresh fruit, oatmeal, soup, whipped cream or stew with your fingers.

*See Recipe section.

8 WAYS FOR A GIRL
to feel lusty

1. Wear heels. They force you to strut!

2. Dress or undress as if your lover is watching you.

3. Skip the underwear, get naughty and go commando on your next date.

4. Wear dangly jewelry, like a necklace that brushes your cleavage or long earrings that tickle your ears or neck.

5. Stand up straight. Walk with confidence and you'll feel that way, too.

6. Wear slinky fabrics. Ditch the sweats and wear something fitted and silky.

7. Use a lubricant. A commercial sex lubricant, such as K-Y or Astroglide, are available at most drugstores and can jump-start a lagging libido.

8. Be a yoga fanatic. Women who practice yoga on a regular basis typically have higher sex drives.

Long Live Lust

Fit people are more sexually active and enjoy sex more than couch potatoes. Additionally, daily relaxation (chronic stress interferes with sexual desire), drinking a little red wine—but not too much—being smart enough not to smoke and maintaining a desirable weight, so that you limit the number of medications you must be on, will go much further in boosting desire, energy and interest than rhino horn, ginseng or oysters. The rest is up to you. Remember—the most important sexual organ and the best aphrodisiac is your imagination.

8

ARE YOU
on the pill?

THE PROMISE

Within **THREE WEEKS** of making these changes, you will

- ✓ Begin lowering your risk for dementia, depression and heart disease.

- ✓ Cope better with stress.

- ✓ Notice improvements in your energy level, if you are a premenopausal woman.

In **SIX MONTHS**, you will

- ✓ Notice continued improvements in memory and thinking.

- ✓ Feel more hopeful and experience more even, positive moods throughout the day.

- ✓ Feel sexier and more "with it."

- ✓ Have more energy.

In **ONE YEAR**, you will

- ✓ Remember where you put your wallet, the pet's name and the name of the last book you read.

- ✓ Feel more yourself, happier and calmer or less agitated.

- ✓ Cope with daily tensions and stress better than you did a year ago.

In **20 YEARS**, you will

- ✓ Think more clearly and remember more than your friends.

- ✓ Be at a lower risk for a host of age-related diseases, from osteoporosis to erectile dysfunction.

I am an absolute believer in taking supplements. Every client who has come to me over the years has been given advice on what to take and how much. I'm not surprised when those clients come back with rave reviews:

- Samantha's energy level improved after she started taking a multivitamin.
- Don swears his memory is better ever since he started taking an omega-3 daily pill.
- Bruce copes better since adding magnesium to his daily supplement routine.
- Carie's depression lifted once she added a multi with folic acid to her day.
- Deb's winter blues are nowhere near as severe since she increased her intake of vitamin D.

As for me, a day without my supplements is a day destined for some unknown health disaster. I just don't feel completely safe without them! The combined effect of eating the S-Ex-Y Diet, plus taking the right supplements and exercising every day must work. I'm over 60 years old, have as much energy and am fitter (and leaner) than I was in my 20s, take no medications, and feel and think great. Of course, I'm not recommending just any ol' supplement. There is more junk than jewels on the market. But take the right ones and I promise you'll see a difference in your mood, memory, energy level and sexy self.

Do You Need the Pill?

 Any of us worth our weight in nutrition credentials will tell you to go to food first for your dietary needs. I agree. Eat a perfect diet and you'll meet almost all your requirements for vitamins, minerals, phytonutrients and fiber. The problem is, close to nobody is eating perfectly. A survey conducted by the U.S. government found that 99 out of every 100 of us don't meet even minimum standards of a balanced diet. We average only three to four servings of fruits and vegetables daily, and even then, choose the absolutely worst options—potatoes, iceberg lettuce and apple juice.

Even if you ate perfectly every day, following the S-Ex-Y Diet guidelines to the letter, your diet probably would come up short for a few nutrients. For example, you would need to drink 10 glasses of milk to get the minimum recommendation for vitamin D and you would far exceed your daily limit for red wine trying to get enough resveratrol. Some nutrients, such as folic acid and vitamin K, are better absorbed or used by the body in supplement form than from food, and other nutrients, such as vitamin B_{12} and calcium, are needed in increasing amounts as we age.

Better yet, compared to people who skip the supplement aisle, those who supplement are typically more health conscious, take better care of themselves, eat better and maintain better overall health, which adds up to whole lot more pizzazz and energy. They also have lower risks for developing heart disease, cancer, osteoporosis, hypertension, memory loss, diabetes, sexual dysfunction, fatigue and birth defects. They have stronger immune systems and are less likely to die prematurely, compared to people who don't supplement.

In short, choosing a great diet and the right supplements is not an either/or issue. You need both. They work together and in tandem. You can't always get optimal amounts of all the vitamins and minerals from food, just as pills don't contain everything that food has to offer. The right supplement plan can replace the handful of vitamins and minerals otherwise found in food, but it never will supply the right balance of the almost 1 million phytonutrients found in authentic foods. No matter what a vegetable-in-a-pill product might promise, you can't freeze-dry, extract, powder or pill all that is in a cornucopia of produce. Period.

On the other hand, you are likely to slip a little from time to time and not eat exactly S-Ex-Y on some days. A good supplement plan can fill in a few of the gaps when you don't eat perfectly. Everyone agrees, however, that supplements n't make up for bad eating habits. You can't live on Ding Dongs and Pop-Tarts, then take a vitamin C supplement and think you're doing fine. But you knew that already, right?

The S-Ex-Y Diet Supplement Plan: The Basics

For healthy people who just want to feel a bit sexier, a multivitamin and -mineral is the place to start. Nutrients are supplied as teams in food, so if your diet is low in one nutrient, it's a sure bet it's low in others, too. A multiple is a convenient, inexpensive way to supply a balance of nutrients, while avoiding secondary deficiencies that result when you take too much of one nutrient and crowd out another. For example, many of the minerals compete for absorption, so taking a large dose of one, such as iron, could result in a deficiency of another, such as copper or zinc. Take a good multi and you won't have to worry about that.

In general, 100–200% of the Daily Value for each nutrient as listed on the Nutrition Facts label is sufficient. Megavitamin-mineral therapy—consuming 10 times or more of the Daily Value—implies that more is better or therapeutic, but usually it's just a waste of money.

Label Lingo

Although the debate rages over which of what is ideal, when it comes to supplements your best bet usually is to stick with the basics and avoid the glitz. Chelated and colloidal minerals are not better absorbed or more potent than other minerals. Time-released vitamins are not well-absorbed and might be more toxic to the liver than a similar amount of a non–time-released brand. Terms such as high-potency, women's formulas or stress-formulated on a supplement are no guarantee of a better formulated product. Natural or organic supplements are no better absorbed and often are a mix of synthetic and natural. (The only exceptions to this rule are with selenium, chromium and vitamin E. The "organic" forms of selenium—selenium-rich yeast or L-selenomethionine and chromium as chromium-rich yeast, chromium nicotinate or chromium picolinate are the best absorbed and used. Body tissues prefer the "natural" form of vitamin E, called d-alpha-tocopherol, to its synthetic counterpart, called dl-alpha- or all-rac-alpha-tocopherol.)

The general rules for choosing a good multi are:

Rule #1 Choose a multiple vitamin-mineral preparation, rather than several single supplements, unless prescribed by a dietitian or nutrition-savy physician.

Rule #2 Choose a preparation that provides 100%, but no more than 300%, of the Daily Value for the following:

Vitamins. Vitamins K, B_1, B_2, B_6 and B_{12}; niacin; folic acid; and pantothenic acid. (Don't be fooled by large doses of vitamin B_1, vitamin B_2 and niacin. A supplement manufacturer adds hefty amounts of these nutrients only because they are inexpensive, not because extra is better.)

Minerals. Copper, iron and zinc, and 50–200 micrograms of both chromium and selenium, 5 milligrams of manganese and 75–250 micrograms of molybdenum.

Rule #3 Vitamins C, D and E can be consumed in amounts greater than the Daily Value. Safe and potentially beneficial amounts of these nutrients are 250–500 milligrams of vitamin C, 1,000–2,000 IU of vitamin D and 100–200 IU of vitamin E. You may need separate supplements to reach these higher doses.

Rule #4 Avoid supplements that contain useless substances, such as inositol, vitamin B_{15}, PABA, or nutrients in amounts less than 25 percent of the Daily Value. The following nutrients are adequately supplied in the diet and are not needed in a supplement:

Biotin   Phosphorus

Chloride   Potassium (if you consume the 9 servings daily of colorful fruits and vegetables)

Sodium

Is it all about Timing?

The time of day has no effect on how well nutrients in a supplement are used by the body. What is more important is what you take them with. Most nutrients are best absorbed when taken with meals. For maximum absorption, take a multiple with iron at a different meal than your calcium supplement, since these two minerals compete for absorption. Also, drink coffee or tea between meals and at a different time than your supplement, since compounds in these beverages, called tannins, block iron absorption.

If you are willing to put up with the inconvenience, select a product that can be taken in several doses. Nutrients supplied in small amounts throughout the day are better absorbed than are one-shot supplements. Multidose multiples also provide flexibility; you can adjust the dose to meet your needs each day.

Gadgets and Gizmos, Bells and Whistles

Vitamins and minerals are basic ingredients, but a well-formulated supplement is a work of art. Nutrients don't just stick together, so manufacturers use binders, stabilizers, fillers and other so-called "inert" substances to make a product that not only stays together in the bottle, but flows through the machinery at the manufacturing plant, protects ingredients from rancidity, keeps a pill from sticking to your throat and makes the tablet or pill a recognizable size. Most of these inert ingredients, including the most common one, calcium phosphate, have safely been used in pharmaceuticals for a long time, so there is no reason to fret. Even the ones that on rare occasions cause side effects, such as FD&C yellow No. 6 dye, lactose or fructose, are unlikely to be a problem at the minuscule doses found in a supplement. For example, the possibility of an allergic reaction to the refined starch used as a filler is extremely rare; the amount of lactose in a supplement is a few milligrams, while it takes grams of lactose to produce a reaction.

Supplement Your Supplement

Most one-pill-a-day multiples don't contain enough of certain minerals. Some nutrients, such as omega-3 DHA, are seldom found in a multi. So there is good reason to supplement your supplement.

Calcium and Magnesium

Bet you can't swallow a golf ball. That's about the size of a supplement containing all the calcium and magnesium you need in a day. Typically, multis give lip service to these nutrients. You need calcium to keep your bones, skin, nerves and muscles in tip-top shape, while magnesium helps you cope with stress, maintain a healthy heartbeat and blood pressure, and strengthen your muscles, nerves and bones. Unless you include at least three servings daily of calcium-rich milk products or fortified soymilk, and lots of magnesium-rich soybeans, nuts and wheat germ, you should supplement these two minerals.

Calcium and magnesium are best absorbed and used when supplied in a 2:1 ratio of calcium to magnesium. You get some of these minerals in your diet, so you only need to fill in the gaps by taking a supplement with about 500 milligrams calcium and 250 milligrams magnesium, if your multiple is low in these minerals. When it comes to magnesium, more is not better. Magnesium is the active ingredient in Milk of Magnesia, which means you could be a bit "looser" than you'd like if you exceed the upper limit of 500–600 milligrams.

The Omega-3s

Having read this far, you probably already are convinced that a day without your omega-3s is a day destined for memory loss, plummeting moods and a heart attack. OK, maybe not quite that dramatic, but the two omega-3s in fatty fish—EPA and DHA—are absolutely critical to mood, mind, memory and sex appeal. If you're not getting at least two servings a week of salmon, mackerel, herring or sardines, and you're not loading foods fortified with an algal-based DHA into your shopping cart and onto your plate, then make sure to take at least 220 milligrams of DHA in pill form; 900 milligrams might be even better.

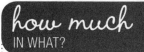

how much
IN WHAT?

A variety of supplements contain a contaminate-free, algal-based DHA. Here are a select few and the amounts per softgel or tablet:

Brain Armor (1,050 mg)	Pure One (300 mg)
Deva Vegan Omega-3 DHA (200 mg)	CVS Algal-900 DHA softgels (300 mg)
BrainStrong Adult (300 mg)	Spectrum Vegetarian DHA (120 mg)
Nature's Way Neuromins (100 mg and 200 mg)	Spring Valley Algal-900 DHA (450 mg)
Ovega-3 (500 mg)	Walgreens Finest Natural–DHA Complete (200 mg)
O-mega-Zen3 (300 mg)	Walgreens Finest Natural Triple Strength DHA Algal-900 (300 mg)
life'sDHA All-Vegetarian softgel (200 mg)	

DO YOU NEED A SUPPLEMENT?

You probably have a pretty good idea whether or not your diet is perfect. But just in case you're still in a quandary as to whether or not to take the pill, here's a quick test to assess what nutrients might be low in your diet.

Do you consume every day:	YES	NO	If "no," your diet could be low in:
1. at least 1 citrus fruit?	☐	☐	Vitamin C, phytonutrients such as limonene.
2. at least 2 dark green leafy vegetables?	☐	☐	Folic acid, vitamin K, iron, calcium, lutein, beta-carotene, etc.
3. at least 9 colorful fruits/vegetables?	☐	☐	B vitamins, trace minerals, 1,000s of phytonutrients.
4. at least 3 glasses of milk, yogurt or fortified soymilk?	☐	☐	Calcium, vitamin D, possibly vitamins B_2 & B_{12}, magnesium, zinc, & probiotics in yogurt.
5. at least 2 servings of extra-lean meat or legumes?	☐	☐	Iron, zinc, B vitamins. Phytonutrients such as phytosterols and saponins in beans.
6. 1 serving of fatty fish?	☐	☐	The omega-3 fats, EPA and DHA.
7. at least 6 servings of whole grains?	☐	☐	Trace minerals, such as chromium, selenium, copper. B vitamins. Phytonutrients such as phytic acid.
8. several servings of nuts, seeds, avocados, olives?	☐	☐	Vitamin E, trace minerals, B vitamins.

Sexy Supplements

Hundreds of supplements, with names like Aroused, Climaxx, Instant Sex, Love in a Jar, Female Virility-V, Maximine's Intima for Women and Libidoblast, promise to put the frisky back into your love life. Most are all promise and no show. Some have scanty research to support the folklore, such as with ayurvedic herbs or roots like Asparagus racemosus, damiana, muira puama, Kali Musli, D-ribose or maca. Others are downright dangerous, especially when they contain ephedra, an amphetamine-like stimulant that won't make you horny, but could keep you up at 4 a.m. shampooing the dog or cleaning the house in a frenzy. At worst, your heart rate could exceed 200 beats/minute, causing dizziness, irregular heartbeat, even death.

The most iffy of all supplements are ones that claim to jack up your hormones, such as testosterone, DHEA (dehydroepiandrosterone) and human growth hormone. Messing with hormones is like playing cards with the devil. The promises are enticing, but the chances of losing are huge. For example, DHEA supplements might increase muscle mass, strength, mood, energy, libido, mental capacity, memory and weight loss, but they also produce unpredictable side effects, ranging from acne and facial hair to liver damage, breast and uterine cancer in women and prostate cancer and aggressiveness in men. No one is even sure how DHEA works in the body, let alone the cost of long-term use. Growth hormone only works when injected and might turn back the hands of time in and out of the bedroom, but it also increases the risk for arthritis, diabetes and hypertension. Men are likely to develop tender, enlarged breasts, while women might be at greater risk for breast cancer.

Other supplements have no credible scientific evidence to support their amorous claims. Black cohosh is supposed to reduce menopause symptoms and reverse vaginal dryness. Dong quai, fenugreek and fennel are supposed to help those who have left lust in the dust. Sorry, Charlie. If any of these work, it is probably because of a placebo effect.

Not only are certain ingredients dangerous, but most are not regulated. As a result, what you think you are buying often isn't what is in the tablet, capsule or pill. In fact, one study found that out of 22 sex-enhancing products, only 9 contained the ingredients listed and were properly labeled.

On the other hand, a few supplements might be worth investigating. The following four pills have reputable research to support their claims. At worst, they are harmless. At best, they might turn the love boat around.

Red Yeast Rice

Supplements of red yeast rice (RYR) are an effective alternative to statin medications in improving blood flow, lowering blood cholesterol levels and reducing heart-disease risk. RYR is made by fermenting yeast (*Monascus purpureus*) over red rice. It contains several active compounds, including monacolins, pigments, fatty acids, trace elements, tannins and other phytochemicals. Compounds in RYR inhibit, by up to 78%, the activity of an enzyme called HMG-CoA reductase, known to increase cholesterol synthesis in the liver. Take RYR and cholesterol synthesis and secretion is dramatically reduced, thus helping prevent and treat high blood cholesterol levels. People who have had a heart attack might reduce their risk of having a second one by up to 45% if they take RYR supplements. In one study, almost 5,000 people with a history of heart attack were randomly assigned to take either placebos or supplements of RYR. At the end of five years, more than 1 in 10 of the placebo group (10%) had experienced another heart attack, compared to only 5.7% of the supplementers, who also were less likely to die from a heart disease problem and were 33% less likely to die from any cause. The need for heart surgery and angioplasty also was lowered by a third.

A word of caution: Researchers at the University of Pennsylvania warn that consumers must be selective in which brand they choose. In their analysis of 12 different brands of RYR, four had detectable levels of a potentially toxic compound, called citrinin, which is produced by a fungus and can damage the kidneys. In addition, the products varied widely in the amount of the active, lipid-lowering compounds, monacolins, with amounts ranging from 0.31 milligrams to 11.15 milligrams per capsule. Levels of monacolin K, also known as lovastatin, ranged from 0.10 to more than 10 milligrams per capsule. Make sure you purchase RYR from a reputable company that guarantees an optimal dose without toxic contamination.

CoEnzyme Q$_{10}$

Every cell in the body depends on a fat-soluble substance called coenzyme Q$_{10}$ (also called ubiquinone or CoQ$_{10}$) to help convert food and oxygen into energy. CoQ$_{10}$ also might help improve heart function, boost immunity and possibly aid in weight management. It is a potent antioxidant, protecting the blood vessels, heart, brain, sex organs and other tissues from free-radical damage. CoQ$_{10}$ even looks promising in extending the healthy years. Typical doses range from 100 to 300 milligrams a day. If you are on statins or even red yeast rice (RYR), make sure you also supplement with this antioxidant, since these medications drain CoQ_{10} from the body.

SAM-e

S-adenosylmethionine (SAM-e) might be even more effective than some antidepressant medications in lifting the depression fog. SAM-e (pronounced "sammy") is made naturally in the body from an amino acid called methionine, along with some help from folic acid and vitamin B_{12}. For some people, the body makes too little of this mood-boosting compound. Supplementing with up to 400 milligrams daily of SAM-e is enough to see major improvements in mood, at least for some people. SAM-e also might be a smart pill, sharpening concentration and accelerating thought processes. A combination of nutrients, including folic acid, vitamin B_{12}, vitamin E and SAM-e, improved quick thinking by up to 20% in one study. There is even some evidence that this little pill might curb Alzheimer's risk. Choose a major brand, like NatureMade, to ensure quality.

Resveratrol

While alcohol might be the greatest aphrodisiac of all time, it is the potent antioxidant resveratrol that might keep you amorous well into your latter years. This polyphenol, found in abundance in red wine, and in lower amounts in red grapes, peanuts, pomegranates and berries, is a potent antioxidant that alters gene expression, turning on cells' production of anti-aging substances. It also speeds cell repair, encourages cancer cells to self-destruct, strengthens blood vessels and lowers the risk for inflammation, heart disease, cancer, dementia, Alzheimer's, menopause symptoms, diabetes and possibly obesity and sexual dysfunction. It even shows promise in extending life span, which means you'll be sexier well into your 90s and beyond. Combining resveratrol with other potent polyphenols, such as those found in curcumin, enhances its potency in fighting disease and aging. There are no guidelines for optimal resveratrol intake, but studies currently are investigating a minimal dose of 20 to 40 milligrams a day, preferably taken in divided doses. (To put this into perspective, a 5-ounce glass of red wine has up to 1.89 milligrams of resveratrol.) You will find supplements that contain much higher amounts, but there is no evidence that high doses produce any greater benefits.

The only glitch here is that resveratrol is best absorbed through the membranes in the mouth, while much of it is broken down in the intestines when taken in pill form. So swish your red wine before swallowing and look for a chewable or dissolvable supplement that lingers in the mouth.

OTHER SUPPLEMENTS THAT
boost sexy

Acetyl-L-Carnitine (Chapter 3)	Huperzine A (Chapter 3)	Saw palmetto (Chapter 6)
Arginine (Chapter 6)	Kava kava (Chapter 2)	Tyrosine (Chapter 3)
Choline (Chapter 3)	Lecithin (Chapter 3)	Valerian (Chapter 2)
Ginkgo biloba (Chapters 2/3)	Melatonin (Chapter 2)	Yohimbine (Chapter 6)
Ginseng (Chapter 2)	Phosphatidyl Serine or PS (Chapter 3)	
Glutathione (Chapter 5)	Pycnogenol (Chapter 5)	

The Whole Story in a Pill

Even the best supplements won't do diddly-squat if you eat junk. However, follow the S-Ex-Y Diet guidelines and combine that diet with a good multi, a calcium-magnesium supplement, a capsule of omega-3 DHA, perhaps some extra vitamin D, and then a sprinkle of the super-sexy pills mentioned above, and I guarantee you'll be saying in no time, "I never knew I could feel this good!"

VITAMINS & MINERALS
at a glance

Here's a brief glance at some of the nutrients needed for health and what you should look for when choosing a supplement.

Nutrient	How much?	Why do you need it?
Vitamin A/ Beta-caro-tene	5,000 IU. Or choose beta-carotene, which is nontoxic at doses of up to 30 milligrams and can be converted to vitamin A in the body. Smokers: Consult a physician before supplementing with beta-carotene since one study found an increased risk for lung cancer in smokers who supplemented with beta-carotene.	Strengthens immunity; maintains healthy epithelial tissues, such as skin, mucous membranes, urinary tract, and the lungs, prostate, vagina and cervix; aids in bone and tooth formation; helps lubricate the vagina and maintain normal vision.
Vitamin D (cholecalcif-erol)	At least 1,000 IU. If blood vitamin D_3 levels are low, you may need 5,000 IU or more. Low vitamin D is defined as less than 75 nanomoles/L of blood.	Aids in calcium absorption and deposition into bones, lowers risk for prostate, pancreatic, breast and colon cancer. Boosts mood and reduces symptoms of seasonal affective disorder (SAD).
Vitamin K (phylloqui-none)	65 micrograms.	Essential for normal blood clotting, helps maintain strong bones, thus reducing osteoporosis risk. Also prevents dark circles under eyes.
Folic Acid	400 micrograms. Don't take more than 800 micrograms without physician approval.	Aids in the growth and development of all normal cells, prevents anemia and birth defects, boosts sperm counts and possibly helps reduce the risk for vaginosis in women, heart disease, age-related memory loss, dementia, depression, cervical dysplasia and colon or cervical cancer.

Continued

Nutrient	How much?	Why do you need it?
Vitamin C (ascorbic acid or calcium ascorbate)	250–500 milligrams are needed to saturate body tissues.	Maintains connective tissue, promotes wound healing, increases iron absorption, strengthens the immune response and, as an antioxidant, prevents damage to tissues, possibly strengthening the body's defenses against cancer, heart disease, high blood pressure, cataracts and other age-related diseases. Might increase frequency and desire for sex, as well as boost mood and help lower stress hormones.
Vitamin E	Doses of 100–400 IU are safe. D-alpha tocopherol is the natural form of vitamin E and appears to be slightly better absorbed by the body than the synthetic dl-alpha tocopherol.	An antioxidant that protects tissues from damage, possibly lowering the risk of developing heart disease, cancer and cataracts. Also strengthens the immune system, aids in blood flow and protects skin from premature aging.
Vitamin B$_6$ (pyridoxine hydrochloride)	2 milligrams. Women on birth control pills might need higher amounts. Excessive doses of 150 milligrams or more might cause tingling in hands and feet.	Aids in the manufacture of all body proteins, including hormones, hormone-like compounds called prostaglandins that regulate blood pressure, enzymes, mood-elevating nerve chemicals, such as serotonin, and hemoglobin in red blood cells. Also aids in muscle contraction and heart function, and strengthens immune response. Might lower heart-disease risk and help prevent memory loss.
Vitamin B$_{12}$	6 micrograms. Older people might need up to 25 micrograms.	Prevents anemia and maintains nerve function, normal cognition and mood-boosting nerve chemical production.
Calcium	1,000 to 1,500 milligrams. Do not exceed 2,500 milligrams. Calcium carbonate and calcium citrate contain the most calcium per tablet. Calcium gluconate or lactate contain less calcium, so more tablets must be taken. "Natural" calcium from oyster shell, bone meal or dolomite often contains lead, a toxic metal.	Reduces the risk of osteoporosis and colon cancer. Aids in blood clotting, blood pressure regulation, muscle contraction and nerve transmission. Might help curb PMS symptoms.

Nutrient	How much?	Why do you need it?
Chromium	Up to 200 micrograms. Chromium nicotinate, chromium-rich yeast and chromium picolinate are absorbed better than chromium chloride.	Aids in blood-sugar regulation. Might lower heart-disease risk.
Copper	2 milligrams.	Aids in nerve transmission and brain function, heart function, red-blood-cell formation and normal hair and skin color. Helps protect cells from damage and assists in blood-sugar regulation.
Iron	Premenopausal girls and women: At least 18 milligrams. Postmenopausal women and men: 10 milligrams. Take iron as ferrous fumarate or ferrous sulfate.	Prevents fatigue, improves exercise performance, strengthens immunity and maintains normal cognition.
Magnesium	About 400 milligrams. More than 600 milligrams might cause diarrhea.	Aids in muscle relation, heart function, nerve transmission, blood pressure regulation, stress reduction, and bone formation and maintenance. Reduces PMS symptoms.
Selenium	Up to 200 micrograms. Selenomethionine or selenium-rich yeast are better absorbed than sodium selenate or selenite.	Reduces tissue damage associated with the development of cancer, heart disease and rheumatoid arthritis.
Zinc	15–25 milligrams. Doses greater than 50 milligrams might suppress immune function.	Aids in wound healing, immune function, the prevention of birth defects and strong bones. Vital for maturing and function of sex glands.

9

CAN YOU SWING
from the
rafters?

THE PROMISE

Within ONE WEEK of making these changes, you will

✓ Notice a boost in energy.

✓ Sleep better (as long as you don't exercise vigorously in the three hours before bedtime).

✓ Possibly drop a pound or two.

✓ Possibly notice an improvement in mood.

Within ONE MONTH, you will

✓ Think faster and remember more.

✓ Feel more confident, vital and sexier.

✓ Lose weight.

✓ Be happier.

✓ Notice that your clothes are a bit baggier.

Within ONE YEAR, you will

✓ Be a whole new you.

✓ Feel 10 years younger.

✓ Look younger.

✓ Be more sexually aroused and enjoy and respond sexually as if you were 10 years younger.

✓ Have lost so much weight you need a new wardrobe.

"I feel frumpy," is how Candice described herself to me at our first session. Recently divorced, she came to me in hopes of "whipping this bod back into shape." After a few months of following my diet advice, she'd dropped a pants size or two, had more energy, slept better and even noticed that her skin had a glow it had lost years ago. But she still wasn't exercising as I'd asked her to do from day one. "I had good intentions to join a gym or dust off the bike, but never seemed to get around to it." After I gave her an ultimatum to either get moving or not bother coming back to see me, she must have realized it was time to get serious.

CAN YOU SWING FROM THE RAFTERS?

Candice took my advice to start her exercise regimen at a crawl. "I set a goal to walk 15 minutes in the evenings. Every week, I upped the ante. First, I picked up the pace, then added a few more minutes, and within two months, I was up to an hour a day of brisk walking. Then I started mixing it up with some biking, too." She dropped weight faster, which motivated her to add a weight training session twice a week to her routine. "I worked out a few times with a personal trainer to learn how to lift right. After that, I bought some weights and did my routine in the living room while watching TV."

Within six months, Candice was a whole new gal. "The diet is so important to how I feel and look, but I have to admit that it was the exercise that really turned on my self-confidence. I've not only lost weight, I've gained a whole new outlook on life." She also reduced, then eliminated, her antidepressants, and left my office medication-free.

> **66** *Exercise is the most important factor in how well you age, in and out of the bedroom.* **99**

Candice is just one of hundreds of people I've known over the years who have confessed that exercise turned their lives around. For example,

- Paisley says, "My mood, energy level, thinking, sleep and coping skills are all directly related to how much I exercise. If I don't exercise I get crabby. It keeps me sane!"

- Lori says, "My daily exercise is empowering. I would be lost without the movement. For me, it promotes creativity and positive feelings."

- Camille says, "I feel most alive when I am dancing, and I see a major difference in my body as a result. My arms have definition and my pooch of a tummy has all but disappeared. I'm just generally more toned and feel good about myself and my body."

- Jerry says, "All my friends are slowing down, complaining about one health problem or another, but I feel better than ever, with all the energy and gusto I had in my 20s. I'm sure that's because I've stayed fit and they've let themselves go."

- Alice says, "My girlfriends sit around and complain about how they have no sex drive, then blame it on menopause, but I'm the oldest one in the group and the only one who exercises every day. I'm hornier than ever!"

- Tony says, "I had a heart attack a few years ago and that was a wake-up call.

I started exercising and eating right after that. OK, it wasn't much fun in the beginning, but within no time, I felt so good—like I'd been given back a 'me' I thought I'd lost—that there is no way I will ever stop exercising!"

- Mark says, "Oh sure, finding time to exercise can be a pain sometimes, but the payoffs make the effort worth it!"

- Tori says, "If I feel my energy dropping midday, I get up and do what I call my 'quickies' for instant energy. I do a minute of jumping jacks and a couple of minutes of running in place, and, wow, I feel like a new woman."

Let's get one thing straight right now. You may feel sexy and cocky in your 20s without doing anything more vigorous than a stroll from the parking lot to the mall, but if you want to stay sexy, sharp, happy and vital after that, you must exercise. (Of course, you'll feel even better in your teens and 20s if you exercise, too!)

Exercise is *the* most important factor in how well you age, in and out of the bedroom. If you don't care enough about your health to exercise regularly, then I hope you have purchased long-term health insurance, because you're setting yourself up for being sick, feeble and frail long before your time. Not to mention the toll being sedentary will take as early as your 40s as your mood, mind, memory, and sex drive and performance plummet.

The Cost of Being Sedentary

> **❝** *Everyone is an athlete. The only difference is that some of us are in training, and some are not.* **❞**
> — George Sheehan, MD

If you don't challenge your muscles with vigorous activity, they start to weaken by your mid-30s. You'll lose about 1–2% of your muscle mass every year after that point, which equates to a 5- to 10-pound loss of muscle every decade. By your 80s (if you make it that far), you will have only a third the muscle mass you had at 40.

As you lose muscle, you gain fat. Metabolism slows with every pound of fat, so you need fewer calories to maintain your weight. Continue to eat like a 20-something and your waistline will expand. Middle-age spread is a clear sign that you are trading muscle for fat, which is a red flag that old age is coming at you like a runaway train. Bones become more porous. Blood pressure, fat and sugar levels rise. You become weaker and more sluggish. The back goes out. Knees hurt. Silently and gradually it takes more effort to do even simple daily tasks; consequently, you do less and less. If you don't stop the process, you will end up on multiple medications, with dementia, and using a walker or a wheelchair.

In short, sloth is the deadliest sin. According to a study from the Cooper Institute for Aerobic Research, the life of a couch potato is at least as risky as a three-pack-a-day cigarette habit. The longer you sit, the shorter your life. It is not a pretty picture, and one that I have no sympathy for, since it is almost entirely preventable. You can set yourself up to be sick or you can choose to be healthy, happy, smart, lean, energetic and sexy. Why would anyone select the former?!

Move It, Baby. Move It!

We are the most unfit humans ever to have walked this planet. It is not natural—although it has become normal—to be sedentary. We are remarkably well-designed over millions of years

ARE YOU *fit?*

You are on the road to Feebleville if you answer "yes" to any of these questions:

- Do you engage in less than 5 hours a week of vigorous, planned exercise?

- Are you out of breath and barely able to talk after bounding up a flight of stairs?

- Are clothes that fit five years ago now too tight?

- Do you avoid bending or stretching because you are too stiff?

- After sitting cross-legged on the floor, does it take a minute or two to loosen up your legs when you stand up?

- Do you find that common household chores, such as washing windows or scrubbing the floor, are more exhausting than they used to be? Are you finding that you avoid doing these tasks as time goes by?

- Can you open a heavy glass door with one hand, or does it require using your body weight?

to be fit. Our ancient hunter-gatherer ancestors were so fit that they ran their game to exhaustion! (Imagine running a deer down?!) Our bodies were meant to move. It is when we don't move, when we don't keep our amazing bodies well-tuned, as Mother Nature designed them to be, that they break down, physically, mentally, emotionally and sexually.

Then there is the weight issue. Even if you are successful at weight loss with the S-Ex-Y Diet alone, you won't maintain that weight loss without exercise. The National Weight Control Registry, which follows thousands of people who have maintained a significant weight loss of 60 pounds or more for at least five years, has found that almost every single one of them exercises regularly.

Exercise also extends life at all ages. People who continue to exercise in their second 50 years are as fit or even fitter than sedentary people who are 20 to 30 years younger, which might explain why they also live longer and healthier, and are most likely to enjoy vigorous sex lives throughout life. The more calories you expend in exercise each week, the longer you are likely to live—and live disease-free.

Move It or Lose It

> **❝** *Out on the roads there is fitness and self-discovery and the persons we were destined to be.* **❞**
> —George Sheehan, MD

Exercise is not just for the body. It's also a major mood and memory enhancer.

Exercise Improves Memory

Exercise reduces inflammation and revs the heart to pump more blood through more capillaries to the brain, along with the rest of the body. Clean, healthy arteries and improved blood flow mean more oxygen, which means better-nourished brain cells. Increased blood flow also raises levels of brain cell–growing factors, such as IGF-1 and BDNF (brain-derived neurotrophic factor), which spark chemicals that increase growth and regeneration of brain cells. BDNF has been called the "Miracle-Gro for your brain." It encourages brain cells to branch out, join together and communicate, which translates into better concentration and learning.

Moderate exercise maintains the brain, while intense exercise grows new brain cells. Even three months of working out daily is enough to sprout new cells in an area of the brain called the hippocampus, where learning and memory take place. At one time, dementia was considered an inevitable consequence of aging, but now researchers recognize that the brain can make new cells, if given a chance. That chance requires daily exercise.

This might explain why physically fit people think more clearly, concentrate better, remember more and react more quickly than sedentary folks. They have less plaque around their brain cells that otherwise would increase the risk for dementia and Alzheimer's disease. They also are leaner, while pudgy couch potatoes are three times more likely to develop dementia as they age.

Exercise Improves Mood

A daily workout amps up brain chemicals, such as dopamine, serotonin, phenylethylamine (PEA), epinephrine and norepinephrine, which boost alertness and focus, improve mood and calm nerves as well, if not better, than antidepressants or tranquilizers. Who wouldn't want to feel better naturally, with no side effects, unless you call feeling great and living healthy longer a problem! Besides, only some people on mood-lifting drugs get full relief—many get no help at all—but everyone benefits from exercise, and often it is the cure. The more you exercise, the lower your risk for depression.

Maybe it's not that exercise is an antidepressant, but rather that *not* exercising is so abnormal to our bodies that it leads to emotional deterioration. In one study, researchers compared the effects of no exercise to various intensities of exercise on psychological outcomes. After 12 months, the sedentary subjects were the ones battling the most stress, anxiety and depression, while the exercisers felt great.

Exercise is a Natural High

Of course, there's also the "exercise high," that burst of euphoria following vigorous activity. This natural high is probably caused by the release of either PEA or the endorphins, the body's natural morphinelike chemicals that help boost pain tolerance and generate feelings of joy and satisfaction. Even a short session, such as a 10-minute brisk walk, is enough for many people to feel just a tad happier. Up the session to 20 minutes of vigorous exercise, such as jumping rope, jogging or aerobic dancing, and that often is enough to rev up sexual appetite.

Exercise is a De-Stressor

If daily worries and stress are messing with your love life, then look to exercise for the cure. Daily activity naturally de-stresses the body by lowering stress hormone levels, including cortisol, that prepare the body for "fight or flight." The rise in body temperature from a vigorous workout has a tranquilizing effect on the body, not unlike soaking in a hot tub, and the increase in blood flow leaves you feeling refreshed and invigorated. Daily exercise also aids sleep. Calm, rested and invigorated...sign me up!

Exercise Lengthens Life

Besides calming nerves and making life today a lot more enjoyable, exercise also extends the healthy years. Stress damages cells by shortening telomeres, the "handles" on the ends of the genetic code, or DNA. Telomeres protect the DNA from fraying and decomposing, but once they are shortened, they can't do their job and the cell self-destructs. It is the accumulation of dead and damaged cells that is a major cause of aging. Vigorous exercise protects telomeres from stress-induced shortening. It is one of the life habits that really and truly extends life!

As Candice found out, exercising every day also is a surefire way to jump-start self-esteem, a sense of accomplishment and feelings of self-control, all of which are strongly linked to being happy and feeling sexy. In fact, study after study finds that people who stick with an exercise program are the most satisfied with their lives in general, and their sex lives in particular.

The Best Aphrodisiac

> 66 *We do not stop exercising because we grow old—we grow old because we stop exercising.* 99
> —Dr. Kenneth Cooper

Being fit dramatically improves your chances of happiness, having more energy, thinking sharply and clearly, remembering more today and down the road, sleeping better, and attaining and maintaining that fit body you've always wanted. You are likely to live longer, are more likely to live disease- and medication-free, look up to 20 years younger and have the most self-esteem, self-confidence and enjoyment in life. It's no wonder you also are likely to feel and look sexier.

Stick with a daily exercise program and you're bound to notice the obvious: more stamina and a slimmer waistline. In contrast, a study published in the *Journal of the American Medical Association* found that people who seldom work out—and that includes sex!—have a much higher chance of suffering a heart attack within two hours of exerting themselves in or out of the bedroom. The more exercise and sex you have, the lower your risk for such problems. What a great reason to get fit in the bedroom. Hey, it takes a lot of energy, speed, flexibility and strength to be a great lover. And the stamina people gain from exercise is the best training session there is!

The link between lust and exercise goes even deeper. The more in touch with your body you are from moving, challenging and using it, the more comfortable and confident you are overall. The increased blood and oxygen flow to tissues means everything works better, from the tip of your head to your lovemaking apparatus. Hormones balance out, testosterone levels rise and men are at much lower risk for erectile dysfunction, while women are hornier, lubricate more readily and have orgasms more often and with more gusto when they are physically fit, no matter what their ages.

Being sexually aroused, whether it is an erection or a lubricated vagina, requires those tissues to swell with blood. While blocked arteries, high blood pressure and other heart-disease issues interfere with those processes, exercise keeps the heart and blood vessels clear and elastic, reducing the risk for any sexual performance problems. The more fit people are, the sexier they feel, the better they respond and the more satisfying their sex lives. Avid exercisers have a "sexual age" that is years younger than their chronological age. Being fit for life means being fit for sex. For example,

- After 20 minutes of aerobic exercise, women are sexually aroused more quickly when viewing erotic films than are women who do no exercise, according to a study from the University of Texas.

- A study conducted at the University of California found that men who worked out three times a week said their sexual performance and frequency of sex improved dramatically.

- Another study found that a high level of sexual activity and satisfaction went hand in hand with being physically fit in both older men and older women.

- Level of physical fitness was directly related to sexual stamina in a study from the University of Medicine and Dentistry of New Jersey, where for every minute of brisk walking on a treadmill, people's sexual stamina improved by 2 minutes.

- A study of 400 women found that those who were physically fit also had the best sex lives.

AGE *accelerators*

Want to age before your time, look forward to dementia and loss of independence, wind up frail and feeble? Here's how to do it:

Shorten telomeres by eating grease, being stressed and not exercising.

Refuse to have an antioxidant orgy, which will increase oxidation.

Weaken the immune system with a pro-inflammatory diet and no exercise.

Pack in the toxins with a highly processed diet, tobacco smoke and smog.

Eat too much junk and be overweight; develop diabetes, high blood pressure and heart disease, for which you require medication.

Upset your neurotransmitter balance with fad diets, skipped meals and being unfit.

Lower nitric oxide levels with too much saturated fat and clogged arteries.

Don't wear sunscreen.

Weaken muscle and brain cells by being sedentary.

In short, the more you move, the better you'll feel, the more energy you'll have, the lower your risk for daily health problems or serious disease, the longer you'll live, and the more you will enjoy sex and the extra years. That is a promise.

So skip the excuses that you're too tired, have no time, are too old, didn't inherit the motivation gene from your grandfather or need to scrub the floors before you can exercise. There is no excuse for not loving yourself enough to take care of the only body and brain you have. Let me repeat—you cannot get to your sexiest self without a daily exercise program.

The S-Ex-Y Fitness Plan

> 66 *There is no substitute for learning to live in our bodies. All the tests and all the machines in the world will fail if we do not first become good animals.* 99
> —George Sheehan, MD

The S-Ex-Y Fitness Plan is as simple as 1, 2, 3: Mix it up at least five days a week with

1 **Aerobic activity** (walking, dancing, rowing, swimming, jogging): Endurance activity strengthens the heart, clears blood vessels, keeps you lean and gives the biggest boost in sexual energy and desire, as well as reduces inflammation and improves mental function and mood.

2 **Strength training** (lifting weights, pilates, calisthenics like situps): Strength training builds muscles that, in turn, improve posture and stamina. It also boosts the metabolic rate, helping your body burn more calories all day long.

3 **Flexibility exercises** (stretching, yoga, tai chi): Flexibility activities enable your joints and muscles to move easily, enhancing every activity, including making it easier to get into your favorite sexual position without fuss, grunts, groans or charley horses.

The foundation of your S-Ex-Y Fitness Plan is the aerobic part, which will strengthen your heart and increase overall blood and oxygen flow. Aerobic activity also is the best way to burn body fat, and it relieves stress.

How do you know if your aerobic exercise is vigorous enough to reap the benefits? By checking your heart rate. Your goal is to exercise within your target heart rate (THR), which is 60–90% of your maximum heart rate (MHR).

1. MHR: subtract your age from 220.
2. THR: multiply your MHR by .60 and again by .90.
   For example, a 45-year-old woman's THR range would be:

   220 – 45 = 175 (MHR)

   175 (MHR) × .60 = 105 beats per minute for 60% of MHR

   175 (MHR) × .90 = 157 beats per minute for 90% of MHR

Take your pulse and monitor your heart rate during exercise by lightly placing your two middle fingers on your throat, just to the side of center, or by placing two fingers on the thumb side of your wrist. Don't press too hard, since this will slow the pulse. Count the beats starting with the number zero on the first beat. Count for ten seconds and then multiply that number by six to determine the total heartbeats per minute. It is important to count the pulse immediately after stopping exercise, since the pulse rate slows quickly once exercise is stopped.

Do occasional spot-checks while exercising. How do you feel when you are working at 40% of your MHR, at 60% and at 90%? How hard are you breathing? Are you comfortable or gasping for air? Are you perspiring? Is your heart pounding wildly or just rhythmically pumping? You want to exercise at a level that allows you to talk and sweat at the same time. If you can't talk, you're exercising too hard and should slow down, even if you're within your THR. If you are within your THR and can sing or whistle while exercising, you are not working hard enough and should increase your exertion to the higher end of the THR scale.

Keep it interesting by mixing up the routine. Rupa walks the dog, takes yoga and also lifts weights. Kim cross-country skis and snowshoes in the winter, and bikes, runs and hikes in the summer. Brenda has lost more than 20% of her body weight by walking on the treadmill and using the spin bike at the gym, then doing aquatic exercises other days or walking the dog. Paisley jumps rope or uses exercise bands some days, then takes yoga, runs or walks other days.

How to Start

> **There are those of us who are always about to live. We are waiting until things change, until there is more time, until we are less tired, until we get a promotion, until we settle down—until, until, until. It always seems as if there is some major event that must occur in our lives before we begin living.**
>
> —George Sheehan, MD

Consider the following before beginning any exercise routine.

- **Get clearance.** If you are over 40 years old, obtain clearance from a physician before beginning an exercise program. Your physician also can help determine at what level you should start the S-Ex-Y Fitness Plan and if there are any undetected health risks that should be considered, such as high cholesterol or blood pressure.

- **Have a plan.** Even if it's something as simple as walking to work, you need to decide how you'll carry your papers or lunch, how you'll keep your work clothes clean and even what route you'll take. You'll also need to purchase the right exercise gear.

- **Expect roadblocks.** Write down all the reasons why you can't exercise, such as can't afford it, no time or don't like to sweat. Next to each, list the reasons why that excuse isn't good enough.

- **Make it the #1 priority.** Before you schedule anything else, set aside a time and place every day for exercise. Don't allow anyone or anything to get in the way. Keep in mind, you will get the same benefits from two to three miniworkouts as long as the total day's time is at least 20 minutes in the beginning and one hour as you become a seasoned exerciser.

- **Set realistic goals.** Vigorous activity is your ultimate goal, but if you haven't exercised in years, you're better off starting slow. That way you're more likely to stick with it than someone who bursts onto the exercise scene with a vengeance. Begin by stretching, walking and doing low-weight strength training. Slowly increase the length of the workout and the intensity. A rule of thumb is to increase the intensity of a workout by no more than 10% each week to reduce the chance of injury (i.e., go from a 3-mile walk one week to a 3.3-mile walk the next week). To see benefits, you must move enough to sweat, but not so much that soreness or fatigue nix your motivation.

- **Define how fit you want to be.** You can't do minimal amounts of exercise and expect major results. Be honest with yourself when matching how much you're willing to move with the weight loss or health benefits you want. If you don't like pain or sweat, then set a moderate pace, but accept that this routine will take more time. For example, you'll need to gradually increase the length of your workouts to at least 90 minutes a day if you want to lose weight. If you want to save time and still shave inches off your waistline, then train harder. The bare minimum is to reach 30 minutes of intense endurance activity four days a week, plus two 20-minute strength training sessions and a few minutes of stretching before and after.

WHAT'S IT *worth*

Just 30 minutes of the following activities will help drop the pounds (assuming you don't increase your intake of doughnuts!):

Activity	Calories	Approximate pounds lost if done every day for 1 month
In-line skating	425	3 ½
Running	374	3
Jumping rope	340	Almost 3
Hula hoop	300	More than 2 ½
Fast dancing	220	Almost 2
Brisk walking	180	More than 1 ½

Vigorous Living

You can get a health benefit from just living, if you do it with gusto. Take the stairs instead of the elevator and walk instead of driving short distances. Walk up the escalator. Get up to change the TV channel. Use a hand-powered can opener. People who increase daily activity lose about the same amount of weight as people who follow traditional aerobic exercise programs. The more they move during the day, the greater the benefits.

Increasing daily activity is as simple as strapping on a pedometer each morning and walking 10,000 steps throughout the day. Be creative and find new ways every day to sneak in the extra mileage, such as walk up and down the hallway when talking on the phone or brushing your teeth. Also, stop using the kids as servants, take miniwalks of one to five minutes several times during the day, use a bathroom on a different floor at work (using the stairs not the elevator to get there), get up to talk to coworkers rather than emailing them, or next time the doctor is running late, use the waiting time to sneak in a 10-minute walk.

Stick with It!

> 66 *A man too busy to take care of his health is like a mechanic too busy to take care of his tools.* 99
> —Spanish proverb

What can you do to avoid skipping the walk the first time it rains? Instead of relying on willpower (aka, self control), I prefer a motivation plan.

Willpower may not be four letters, but it is still a dirty word, and seldom comes through when you need it most. But, focusing on the positive by having a motivation plan can build willpower and help you resist the temptation to buy fresh-baked goodies when passing Cinnabon at the mall or to give in to the excuse that you are just too tired to work out.

First, keep in mind that even those born with no backbone can develop self-control. Practice makes perfect, even in the game of willpower. Think of building willpower just as you build muscle. It may hurt at first, but with repeated practice, the effort develops into a habit. You are most likely to be successful if you build your willpower muscle gradually by setting realistic goals that start small and grow big over time. Like Candice, start by walking 15 minutes, three days a week. Then have a specific plan as how to gradually increase the intensity, time and frequency over the next six months.

Enforce the "if…then" rule. Decide on a motivating reward system that works for you. Perhaps it is stars on a calendar or money in a jar every time you exercise, which then goes toward a new outfit or seeing a special movie. *If* you exercise, *then* you get the star or money. No exercise, no star. If you find yourself slipping, then the reward isn't working and you need to find one that is more motivating.

Trick yourself. I have been exercising vigorously for more than 35 years and I still need to trick myself into doing it. I find every excuse in the world why I can't drive the half hour to the gym to lift weights. So for me it is worth it to have a personal trainer who demands that I show up three days a week. Here are other ways to trick yourself into exercising:

- Tanya calls her friends on Sunday night to schedule walking dates throughout the week. "I have to show up because they are expecting me to be there," she notes.

- Paisley says, "I motivate myself to cycle by reminding myself that if I was physically challenged and couldn't ride, I would yearn for the blessing of being physically active. I ride because I *can*!"

- Sally says, "I can't stay on the exercise bicycle for more than 15 minutes at home without the irresistible urge to unload the dishwasher or wash the sheets. But if I pedal to a musical, like *Chicago* or *Mamma Mia!,* cycling like a madwoman during the songs and sanely during the talking parts, I can stay on the bike for a full hour."

- Sam made a bet with his best friend that he could lose the most weight and be the fittest within one year. "I love a competition and you'd better believe that even on nights when I want to collapse in the recliner, all I have to do is remind myself that Hank is probably working out right now, and I am on it, in my sweats and headed for a workout."

Pre-Workout Quickies

> 66 *Take care of your body. It's the only place you have to live.* 99
>
> —Jim Rohn

Just because you went for a 10-minute walk for the first time in five years, doesn't give you permission to eat a Big Mac for lunch! Your calorie intake won't need a shot in the arm until you are exercising vigorously and daily for at least 45 minutes. But once you have made the S-Ex-Y Fitness Plan a habit, then you may need to think about a Quickie snack before you hit the road or gym.

The goal of a preworkout Quickie snack is to stay hydrated and maintain a constant glucose source for the muscles, so you don't dip too far into your reserves—the glycogen stores. To meet this goal, a preworkout snack should include water and quality carbs, since carbs—from pasta to pretzels—are merely long strings of glucose molecules. Go for snacks (and your diet overall, for that matter) that are about 60% carbs, since this is the level of carb intake that maximizes glycogen storage. However, carbs alone, especially sugary ones, such as sweetened sports drinks, can cause blood sugar to nosedive midworkout. A bit of protein from yogurt, milk, soymilk or nuts offsets this drop, helps shuttle carbs into muscle cells where they are needed most and aids in repairing and building muscle. This carb-protein snack should be low-fat and light—say, 100 to 300 calories—to avoid digestive problems. (Blood supply to the digestive tract drops up to 80% during a workout, which can cause indigestion if there's food lingering in the stomach.) The size of the snack varies from person to person, so it's best to err on the side of caution by eating less at first and then make adjustments as you go. Along with your water bottle, easy-to-digest Quickie snacks include:

Half a whole-wheat bagel with a little low-fat cheese.

A soft whole-grain pretzel with nonfat yogurt.

Whole-wheat toast, topped with apple butter and fat-free cottage cheese.

Small helpings of leftover rice or pasta dishes.

A small slice of last-night's vegetarian pizza *(such as Passionate Peppered Pizza or Ya' Wanna Pizza Me! in the Recipe section)*.

A small helping of Seriously Sensuous Honeyed Fig Oatmeal *(in the Recipe section)*.

String cheese with apples and whole-grain crackers.

A small bowl of whole-grain cereal with light soymilk.

Timing is important. Plan to snack one to two hours before a workout to enhance performance without upsetting your stomach. Liquids are digested faster than solids, so an 8-ounce fruit and yogurt smoothie or a glass of nonfat milk might be the best bet for a snack in the hour before a run or any bouncy sport. Have a bigger meal but allow more time—up to four hours—before jumping into a heavy-duty workout, to ensure that food has emptied from the stomach and is at least partially digested. If that hefty workout is at 6 a.m., have something light, such as a few graham crackers, as you head out the door for a 6-mile run.

The right snack can curb hunger and provide the energy needed to enjoy a workout, which is a motivator to exercise more often. However, it's only part of an overall high-performance diet, and won't make up for not following the S-Ex-Y Diet guidelines, such as skipping breakfast or living on coffee through lunch. It's what you've eaten all day, starting with breakfast, that will make or break not only your workout, but also your overall health and vitality.

The S-Ex-Y Fitness Plan: Little Pain, Huge Gain

The road to sexy is paved with exercise. It arouses the body, sharpens the senses, increases blood flow to tissues including the brain and sex organs, pumps oxygen to every tissue, lowers stress, improves sleep, builds self-confidence, kick-starts lusty appetites, slims the waistline, reduces the risk for all age-related diseases and extends the healthy years. Incorporate the three-step S-Ex-Y Fitness Plan into your daily routine and I promise you will be swinging from the rafters with a grin on your face in no time!

> **❝** *If you don't know where you are going, you will wind up somewhere else!* **❞**
> —Yogi Berra

10

DO YOU EMBRACE
sexy habits?

THE PROMISE

Within ONE WEEK of making these changes, you will

- ✓ Begin to build new brain pathways. This increased Brain Reserve will pay off with better memory and lower dementia risk later in life.
- ✓ Notice a slight improvement in thinking ability.

In ONE MONTH, you will

- ✓ Have found more purpose in life.
- ✓ Feel more alive.
- ✓ Be more grateful.
- ✓ Think more clearly.
- ✓ Be calmer and less stressed.

In ONE YEAR, you will

- ✓ Be happier with yourself and your life.
- ✓ Feel sexier.
- ✓ Think more positively and hopeful.
- ✓ Be at lower risk for disease, dementia and depression.
- ✓ Be more fun to be around!

"You weren't born to be depressed, forgetful or frumpy. All of these are huge red flags that your life is out of balance and your spirit is out of whack," I told Susan, who sat slumped, exhausted and on the verge of tears in my office. She came looking for nutrition advice, which I was glad to give, but I suspected that there was more to her problem than just the need for a diet makeover.

Susan was a working mom with a husband who did little to help. "I'm racing from the time my feet hit the floor until the moment I collapse in bed at night," she admitted. It is difficult to feel sexy if you're living a frantic life, one that gives you no time to connect with your inner sexy, or one not in tune with who you really are. This was a perfect opportunity for Susan to step back; take a good, long look at what was draining her life spirit; and then plot a course toward a new, better and sexier self.

The road to a fit and sexy body and mind is not paved with diet and exercise alone. Even if you follow the S-Ex-Y Diet and Fitness Plan to the letter, you still are feeding your brain junk and depleting your energy if the rest of the day is packed with unstimulating, sluggish or downright exhausting errands, busywork, people and routines.

How you spend your time says much more about you than anything you might say is your priority. Susan said her health was second only to her family, yet her days were a race to pack lunches, get the kids to school, work, shop, shuttle kids to piano lessons, make dinner, give baths, do housecleaning and finish up work from the office. The occasional free moment was spent comatose in front of the television. There was little "health" in the details of her day. Her stressed-out schedule meant she had lost touch with friends, no longer went to her book club meetings and had given up her favorite hobbies of gardening and photography. In the rush to get everything done, she'd misplaced her curiosity, adventuresome spirit and openness to life, while her sexy self had drained out along the way.

I didn't want to overwhelm Susan with a total life makeover right away, so we started slow. I gave her ideas for healthy meals and Quickie snacks, and she promised to exercise, if only for 10 minutes a day. Over the following weeks, Susan and I fine-tuned her diet and developed a workable plan for more exercise. As her energy level improved and her mind sharpened, she was motivated to take on other aspects of her life. It didn't take long and it did take some work, but the payoffs made the effort worth it. By the time Susan left my office for the last time, she had lost 30 pounds, was training to run her first 10K race, had more time for fun with family and friends, and was feeling sexy and alive again.

Like Susan, most of us could use an occasional life review. Every decision we make, every choice we have from minute to minute, either increases our chances of happiness or drains a bit away. That sharp mind, glowing skin, vibrancy and good mood today, and sharp-as-a-tack mind down the road, are to a great extent the results of living well now. But often, days, months, years, even decades go by without a break in the mayhem to evaluate whether we are even enjoying our lives, let alone if those lives are good for us.

Make a few changes in your approach to life and how you choose to spend your time, and you will notice something akin to a miracle in your happiness. Are you choosing sexy or are you choosing frumpy? Let's see.

Cop a Sexy Attitude

> 66 *Attitude is more important than the past, than education, than money, than circumstances, than what people do or say. It is more important than appearance, giftedness or skill.* 99
>
> —W. C. Fields

It wasn't the *Mona Lisa,* but it was in Paris that I learned my first lesson about smiling. I was having dinner with the French artist who had sketched my portrait that day in Montmartre. I must have been as animated then as I am now, with my arms and hands flying about and a face miming every emotion, because at some point my new artist friend leaned across the table and warned me that if I continued to smile so much, I would end up a wrinkled old lady. I was only 18 years old, impressionable and naive, but I knew enough to shoot back, "I would choose wrinkles any day over a life without laughter and smiles!" Easy enough to say when you are a teenager, with a blank slate for a face, yet for once in my life, I was wiser than my years.

When it comes to sexy, attitude is everything. People with sunnier outlooks on life age well, live longer (more than seven years on average, according to a study from Yale) and have lower rates of disease throughout life. They recover from surgery faster, have lower heart-disease risks, are in better physical health, have more vitality and suffer less pain than do curmudgeons. Laughter also reduces inflammation and depression, and kick-starts the immune system.

Upbeat thinking also begets more happiness. Every time you think positive, it changes your brain chemistry, with higher levels of feel-good chemicals, such as dopamine and the endorphins. An upward spiral results where the improved brain function further encourages a happier outlook. (Negative thoughts have just the opposite effect, creating a spiral of negative thoughts that kill brain cells and squelch happiness and healing.) The health benefits are strong, but transient, so refuel regularly with smiles and laughter throughout the day.

Don't get me wrong. I'm not suggesting that you ignore pain or deny your problems. Just put them in perspective. Bad things happen to everyone, whether you are a Pollyanna or a Scrooge. Life hurts sometimes. But the Pollyanna bounces back faster and suffers less from the damaging effects of stress and depression. As

Dr. Dan Baker says in his book, *What Happy People Know*, "Happiness isn't the art of building a trouble-free life. It's the art of responding well when trouble strikes." You can't avoid problems, hardships, even crises, but you can nurture a life that helps you cope and returns you to sexy as soon as possible. That means ignoring the advice of that French artist and adopting an optimistic attitude. Scrunch up your face with a smile!

Tricks of the Happiness Trade

Health is sexy, and sexy is all about cherishing every day. It's about love, humor, health, being optimistic, having a purpose, feeling secure, giving and being kind to others. To nurture this, you must work at it, just as you would work out your muscles with exercise. You can't expect to be fit by thinking about exercise. You also can't expect to be fully happy and sexy by just thinking about it. Besides, it takes just as much effort to be happy as it does to be crabby, so put your energy where it will help, not hurt!

When you don't feel happy, act "as if" you are. In other words, fake it 'til you make it. Put on a happy face, walk tall and shut out the killjoy thoughts, worries and frets long enough to be kind to those around you. Share happy memories, connect with people by looking them in the eye. Say "thank you" a hundred times a day and mean it! Even if you don't feel sexy, slap on a smile and greet people with a face full of welcome. You'll get more smiles back, which will help you feel better. And studies show that men find women more attractive when they radiate confidence.

> **"** *...focus on your possibilities, strengths and assets...* **"**

Sexy springs from the thoughts you choose to harbor. Choose nurturing thoughts that are playful and positive, and you take one step at a time toward feeling vibrant. On the other hand, choose to nurture negative thoughts with words like *I can't* or *I shouldn't,* and you quickly turn into your own worst enemy when it comes to finding inner happiness. Give up the excuses that foster negative thoughts, like these: You have no power or control (the "Poor me. Why me?" attitude), you deserve more of this or that, you are waiting for someone to take care of you or some aspect of your life ("Once I find a wife/husband/job/etc., my life will be complete") or you blame someone or something for where you are ("I had a hard childhood, no wonder I'm overweight"). Choose your strengths, not your weaknesses, and use those to fashion your thoughts.

If you think this is a lot of work, tough. Anything worth having is worth working for, right? Besides, without effort, you are likely to feel weak and worthless. You'd be just a leaf in the wind. Make the effort and take charge of your attitude every moment, focus on your possibilities, strengths and assets, and get going on the road to sexy! It will attract love.

An Attitude of Gratitude

Adopting an attitude of gratitude is one of the fastest ways to wrap yourself in happiness. One study from the University of California at Davis divided hundreds of people into three groups and asked each group to keep a journal. One group wrote down daily events, the second group monitored their daily hassles and the third group listed every day the things they were grateful for. At the end of the study, which group do you think was most alert, happiest and felt most loved? You got it. The group who focused on what they had, not what they didn't have, was the one with the best attitude.

How do you nurture gratitude? Throughout the day, schedule four or more 30-second stops in which you close your eyes, relax and take time to be grateful for all you have. Even visualize yourself joyful. Or try keeping a gratitude journal. Every night before you turn out the light, write down five things you are grateful for that you haven't listed in at least a year. This simple habit will strengthen optimistic thoughts. Better yet, it becomes a great resource to look back on in times of trial. You will find that you are literally overwhelmed with how many wonderful things you have in your life!

Use It or Lose It

> 66 *You must begin to think of yourself as becoming the person you want to be.* 99
>
> —David Viscott

My daughter stood in the doorway staring at me with a concerned look on her face. "Mom, what in the world are you doing?" She'd caught me in the midst of one of my many quirks. I was writing my name backwards. She must have thought I was headed for the loony bin.

Shh. Don't tell anyone, but I also sometimes brush my teeth or eat with my left hand (I'm right-handed), walk backwards while tossing a ball, refuse to use a GPS so frequently and intentionally get lost, close my eyes and walk around the house, and typically pop in my Italian tapes rather than music when I'm driving. There is a method to this madness.

Left unstimulated, the brain slips into sluggish thinking. Every time you do something out of habit or choose the predictable, your mind switches to autopilot. The more routine your life and the less stimulating, the faster brain cells deteriorate and the higher your risk for memory loss today and dementia down the road. That explains why people who watch more than an hour a day of television also are the ones most prone to heart disease and dementia. They don't call it the "boob tube" for nothing!

Your brain starts its nosedive into Forgetville as early as the mid-20s. But, keep learning and you stimulate connections between brain cells and increase their numbers, which gives you a greater Brain Reserve. You can keep that noggin of yours running at peak performance and even make improvements at any age. Just like the body, you can "use it or lose it."

Brain Reserve 101

The term *Brain Reserve* refers to the brain's ability to physically reorganize itself in response to the demands placed upon it. A brain with a strong Reserve is one that has formed many

> **"** *The older and sharper you get, the healthier you and your life choices have been.* **"**

cell connections and is rich in brain-cell density, with lots of alternative cell pathways that compensate for any local damage. Think of it as having more than one road to your destination, which allows you to get there even if some roads are blocked.

The best example of how to build an ample Brain Reserve is the famous Nun Study. In 1986, elderly members of the School Sisters of Notre Dame began participating in this study on aging. They agreed to yearly tests of their mental and physical functions, a variety of medical tests and the donation of their brains upon their death. Results found that the more highly educated the nuns were, the fewer symptoms of cognitive decline they showed. The nuns who had a better grasp of language in early life were less prone to dementia, and those whose early writings revealed a positive outlook lived longer than those who didn't. The best of all was the astounding Sister Mary who, at the age of 101, showed no signs or symptoms of mental frailty—even though the autopsy of her brain revealed the structural changes usually associated with advanced Alzheimer's. Wow!

What can we take away from this study? People who stay mentally stimulated, with greater vocabularies and mental challenges, are the ones most likely to remain dementia-free throughout life. Even if some of their brain cells are diving into chaos, there is enough Reserve to compensate. They may have the disease, but they have developed ample alternate routes to continue thinking clearly, quickly and creatively.

The sooner you start building your Brain Reserve, the better and sexier you'll be today and for the rest of your life. The more alert, educated, mentally stimulated and active you are and the sooner and younger you start, the longer you will live mentally vibrant. In short, the older and sharper you get, the healthier you and your life choices have been.

Build a Better Brain

My mom died from complications of Alzheimer's disease. You'd better believe that I am doing everything possible not to follow in her footsteps. Every day I challenge my mind. I stick to the S-Ex-Y Diet guidelines. I exercise at least six hours a week, usually more. I challenge my brain with puzzles, learning Italian, getting lost so I have to figure out how to find my way . . . you name it.

You will choose an entirely different set of brainteasers. You might learn sign language, play a violin, do needlepoint, learn to juggle, assemble furniture, visit an aquarium, use your imagination or play chess, checkers, bridge, backgammon or pinball. Even dancing with your partner can help, since it combines physical activity, socializing and mental challenge. I don't care what you do, as long as you turn off the boob tube and undertake a variety of challenges every day that jolt the brain and encourage it to build, not break down, its Brain Reserve. Besides, you will be much more attractive and interesting if your life is, too.

Happy Friends

I hope that by now I've convinced you that a fundamental quality of sexy is happiness. Not as in living in la la land, but the true joy that comes from feeling good about yourself, being

> **❝** *Friendship is a single soul dwelling in two bodies.* **❞**
> —Aristotle

comfortable in your own skin and at peace with your life. The foundation of that happiness comes from taking care of yourself by feeding the body and brain with the building blocks it needs to think clearly and produce feel-good chemicals, as well as daily exercise that enhances those brain chemicals and flushes out toxins that otherwise undermine mood. Once you are following the S-Ex-Y Diet and Fitness Plan, can you guess the next aspect of your life that has the biggest benefit for happiness?

If you guessed money, you're wrong. Studies repeatedly find that once people have their basic needs met for food, shelter and clothing, additional money does not bring any more happiness. The average American is twice as rich compared to 40 years ago, but is no happier and is 10 times more likely to be depressed.

If you guessed possessions, such as a new house, a plane, a fancy car, the latest designer jeans or a Droid, once again you are wrong. Acquiring the possession is fun, but people typically are no more happy once they have whatever it was they thought they wanted. If you guessed power, you're wrong, too. You never have enough, so the more power and status people accumulate, the more insecure they are about losing it, and the more they want. The correct answer is a loving network of family and friends.

It makes sense. We are tribal, clannish, herd animals by nature. We evolved living and depending on a close community for survival. Being part of a supportive clan—whether it is Susan's book club or your church group—reduces depression and suicide risk, and alcohol abuse. Volunteering also works. You are most likely to live longer (up to 30% longer), have more energy, recover from illness faster, lower your stress and have a greater sense of control over your life if you are connected to and helping out a supportive tribe. It gives purpose and meaning to life, and increases overall life satisfaction as well as sexual satisfaction. You will lower your risk for heart disease and high blood pressure, too!

Of course, you can't plop yourself at church and expect a miracle. Pleasure is a crucial factor in brain health and mood. You must enjoy what you're doing for it to work. So choose a group activity that dovetails with your beliefs and values. If you don't have time to volunteer at your church, humane society or other organizations in town, then help out a neighbor, friend or family member every chance you get.

Susan had traded her social network for a "to do" list. It was absolutely critical to her happiness that she rearrange her life so that the girlfriends in her book club and the neighbors she loved could be part of her life again. This meant a heart-to-heart with her husband. "I told him our marriage was on the line and I needed him to either start participating in family chores or cough up more money so I could hire a maid, gardener and part-time nanny," she told me. He chose the former and they came up with a plan where he took over at least part of his share of the child-care and household duties, which freed up her time to rejoin her book club, as well as exercise and write in her journal.

Who's Minding the Store?

> 66 *Eighty percent of success is showing up.* 99
> —Woody Allen

Pay attention. That seems like obvious advice, but how many of us stumble through the day on autopilot, only half aware of what is going on? We rush through things without being fully attentive. We don't notice subtle signs of tension or stress. We nibble without being aware that we are eating. We find ourselves thinking more about the next task instead of the one we are doing. We forget a person's name as soon as we hear it. All of that is mindlessness.

The more alert we stay, the more active our minds and the more we enjoy each moment. It's called *mindfulness,* and studies show that being truly aware and in the moment throughout the day increases sexual response, reduces sexual anxiety, bolsters positive thoughts, lowers stress and increases life expectancy. One study from Wake Forest University School of Medicine found that even four days of practicing mindfulness was enough to see significant improvements in thinking.

There is a basketful of techniques to encourage mindfulness, but the best one is meditation, which increases awareness, attention span and memory, while improving energy, vitality, self-control and empowerment, and lowering insomnia and disease risk. Studies show that people who are typically happy and calm show the greatest activity in the left side of their brains' frontal area, while people who harbor negative thoughts and are more prone to depression have more activity on the right side of their brains' frontal area. Meditation shifts this "emotional set point" in favor of happiness. In short, even if you were born a grump, you can tweak the circuitry toward happy, calm and sexy by choosing the right habits and hobbies.

Mindfulness can be embraced anytime, anywhere. Sit comfortably with your eyes closed in a quiet place. Breathe slowly and let your muscles relax. Then repeat a phrase, word, or sound—maybe even a short prayer—over and over for a few minutes, while ignoring other thoughts. Open your eyes and get on with the day, reminding yourself from time to time to *pay attention!* If you feel guilty doing nothing but meditating, remind yourself that you are busy lowering your stress hormones and saving brain cells. It is a gift to your mind!

Other ways to calm down, protect brain cells and be more mindful include acupuncture, biofeedback, yoga and massage. These relaxation habits reduce stress and depression, lower cortisol levels and even improve your sex life. Biofeedback also allows you to control blood flow, reduce migraine headaches and control the stress response. Scented massage oils, such as jasmine oil, not only relax you, but also stimulate arousal, so you get a one-two punch for feeling sexy. Even increasing the amount of time you spend in the sun can elevate your mood. So open the drapes and let the light stream in. If you live in an area that is gloomy, buy a biolight and sit in front of it for a few moments in the morning. It will perk you up.

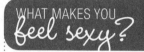

WHAT MAKES YOU feel sexy?

Find your true sexy self every day by answering the following questions:

- What do you like the most about yourself?

- What are your strong points? What nurtures these qualities?

- When do you feel your best? What can you do to make that feeling last longer?

- When do you feel most confident? What is going on? Who are you with?

- Who brings out the best in you?

- What makes you feel sexy?

- When did you feel your sexiest? What contributed to your feeling sexy then?

- What can you do today to feel more confident and sexy?

Do This, Not That

66 *Running is the greatest metaphor for life, because you get out of it what you put into it.* 99
—Oprah Winfrey

Eat right, move more, be kind, think positive, help others, challenge your brain, pay attention. All these habits boost your sexy quotient, no matter what your age. It's important to include things in your life that make you feel good and sexy. That will vary from person to person, so take some time to think about when you felt your sexiest and why. Then add more of that back into your life. For example,

- Camille says, "Wearing stylish, slim-fitting clothes makes me feel sexy, gives me confidence and makes me feel successful. I also feel my sexiest over a meal by candlelight with soft music, an elegant table, intimate conversation over a meal served in courses, slowly with no sense of time and, of course, exquisite red wine and sparkling water."

- Rupa says, "Dressing well, fixing myself up and smiling make me feel good about myself. I like to be noticed by people. I find people smile because I smile at them."

- Kim says, "When did I feel my sexiest? Well, a memory that comes immediately to mind is our first date. Oysters and martinis. It was pretty sexy!!! We didn't actually have sex that night, but our son wasn't too far behind!"

- Jim says, "I used to play the guitar, but with my busy life, I'd put that hobby aside. I just picked it up the other day and found it gave me so much satisfaction and helped me relax. I plan to play on a regular basis from now on."

- Brenda says, "Definitely losing weight has made a big difference in how I feel about myself. I walk taller and sleep better. I look in the mirror and now see someone I like. Before, I would avoid the mirror and hated getting up in the mornings to brush my hair and teeth."

- Jared says, "I feel on top of my game when I work out regularly. I walk taller, feel better, and that seems to attract more women, too. I also love spending time hiking in the woods. It seems to center me and helps me appreciate all that I have in the rest of my life."

- Grace says, "It took me a long time, but I finally found a purpose in life that really makes me feel grounded and happy. I recently was certified as an emergency medical technician (EMT). Now I volunteer at the free clinic on my days off."

- Paisley says, "I feel the happiest when I'm busy. I love to see the calendar filled with work, activities, get-togethers with friends and family. On slow days, I volunteer at the wildlife rescue center. I also love to try new things, especially things I never would or could do before."

There are a few habits you also don't need. Anything having to do with tobacco is an absolute no-no when it comes to sexy. Tobacco kills with every inhale. It reduces sperm counts, volume, mobility and vitality, while undermining sexual function and increasing the chances of sexual problems. And while a glass of red wine at night is a great aphrodisiac, too much alcohol turns a lover into a loser and accelerates brain-cell death.

Ironically, not having enough sex also can undermine happiness. People who have a satisfying sex life tend to be happier than people who abstain. They also are healthier and live longer. Some experts even go so far as to recommend sex as medicine to improve overall health. Of course, desire stems from being healthy, having a good relationship with your partner—in and out of the bedroom—a healthy self-esteem and good feelings about your body. Following the S-Ex-Y Diet and Fitness Program, while building a happy life, provides the building blocks for great sex.

Shine, It's Sexy

66 *There is a vitality, a life force, an energy, a quickening, that is translated through you into action, and because there is only one of you in all time, this expression is unique.* 99
—Martha Graham

Sexy is an attitude and a lifestyle. You either choose to work at being sexy or you choose to work at being less than you can be. The effort is the same. Looking sexy, feeling sexy, being sexy—it's all about radiating an inner health and beauty. It lies much deeper within you than just the clothes you wear, the house you live in or the job you have.

Sexy is feeling confident, having a purpose and meaning in life, living true to your values and passions, and being a giving, caring member of a supportive community. It requires eating well and being physically active, mentally engaged and socially connected. Your body and brain require optimal nourishment from the S-Ex-Y Diet, a daily invigorating workout from the S-Ex-Y Fitness Plan, and ample sleep, low stress and good health habits.

You also are a spirit. The spirit shines when you nourish and care for the house your spirit lives in (that would be your body). It shines when nourished with gratitude, habits that foster contentment and happiness, and finding time each day to give and be kind. A spirit that shines is the ultimate SEXY!

part
TWO

THE GET-SEXY
daily planner

Congratulations!

You've read the "get sexy" plan from cover to cover. You've reviewed the tips, tricks, recommended habits and remedies that absolutely will help you become even happier, leaner, smarter and sexier than you ever have been before. Now what?

Where do you begin to transform yourself from good to great? How do you put know-how information into can-do practice? How do you turn a book of tips into an as-natural-as-taking-a-breath habit?

The following daily planner is the ultimate, get-sexy hour-by-hour daily routine. It is designed merely as a guide, a sample day. Tweak, adapt, adjust, personalize as you and your life demand, based on the hundreds of tips and pieces of advice offered throughout this book.

In general, the following perfect day is based on the fundamentals of the S-Ex-Y Diet and Fitness Plan. Every day

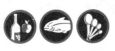

1. Aim for a diet where 75% of the foods are authentic, nonprocessed foods. That means every plate should be piled high with colorful fruits and vegetables, whole grains, omega-3 DHA-rich foods such as salmon, legumes, nuts and other real food. Less-healthy foods—the remaining 25% of the diet—can be more processed stuff, but that should be seriously limited in portions and frequency.

2. Eat regularly, starting with the Ménage à Trois breakfast, followed by Quickie or G-Spot snacks, a Twosome lunch and a light dinner.

3. Take your supplements, such as a multi, a calcium-magnesium supplement, and omega-3 DHA, with meals.

4. Exercise, mixing and matching the 1, 2, 3 S-Ex-Y Fitness Plan of aerobic, weight strengthening and flexibility exercises.

5. Live sexy. Actively decide that you want to take care of yourself, be happy and feel sexy. Stay social, read, play mind-provoking games, volunteer, pay attention, relax, keep a gratitude journal and/or join a group, such as a church or book club.

Here's how to put that plan into action.

6:30 a.m.*

Wake up after 7 or 8 hours of restful sleep, feeling refreshed and ready for the day.

Do some gentle stretching or a few yoga moves, such as sun salutations. Exercise for 20 to 60 minutes now or later in the day. Make coffee or tea, take a shower, apply moisturizer over your body and a cream or gel with age-defying AHAs to smooth fine lines and wrinkles. Apply sunscreen. Weigh yourself to catch any small gains in weight. Choose an outfit that makes you feel confident. Breathe and remind yourself to *pay attention* throughout the day.

7:15 a.m.

Have a Ménage à Trois breakfast. Take your supplements. Pack one or two Quickie snacks, a water bottle, and a Twosome lunch. If you work, take those with you. If you are getting the kids off to school or running errands, put the lunch in the fridge and bring snacks and water with you.

7:50 a.m.

Take a few minutes to organize your day. Make a list of what you can realistically accomplish, write your grocery list, if necessary. Remind yourself of your goals for the day, such as to stand up straight, greet people with a smile, think positively, be kind and grateful, breathe.

8:00 a.m.

Brush teeth, adjust clothes, apply makeup, style hair, etc. Women— do Kegel exercises (squeeze the muscles that control urine flow and hold for a count of 5, relax and repeat five times) in the car. The more of these you do throughout the day, the better will be your love life.

---

*These times are arbitrary and depend on your schedule, lifestyle and preferences.

10:00 a.m.

Take a break. Walk for 5 minutes or do some stretching exercises. Have a cup of green tea and a Quickie snack if you feel a bit hungry. Go outside and breathe fresh air for a minute. Shake off any stress. Take a moment to compliment a coworker or friend.

11:15 a.m.

Get up and walk around, stretch, touch your toes. Smile.

12:15 p.m.

Lunchtime. Pull out your Twosome brown bag lunch, sit back and slowly and consciously enjoy every bite while relaxing and perhaps visiting with coworkers or a friend. Then, go for a brisk 15-minute walk. Reapply sunscreen, if necessary. Drink a glass of water upon returning from the walk. Remind yourself of your goals for today. Breathe, smile and *pay attention.*

1:30 p.m.

Get up and walk around, stretch, do some jumping jacks. Smile.

3:30 p.m.

Have a Quickie snack. Drink water. Get up and walk, stretch or climb stairs for 5 minutes.

5:15 p.m.

Exercise if you didn't in the morning. Or meditate, volunteer or spend time with a friend.

6:30 p.m.

Have a glass of water while preparing dinner with your partner. Don't mindlessly taste-test. (Every bite packs about 25 calories. Four mindless bites while cooking adds up to a 1-pound weight gain by the end of the month.) Women—do more Kegels during your evening routine. Sit at the table with family and/or friends if possible, and have a light, low-fat meal. Light candles, set the table and make the experience soothing and one that encourages conversation. Take any remaining supplements that were not taken at breakfast.

7:30 p.m.

Brain Reserve time: Go to your book club, do Sudoku, play Scrabble or be active, such as ride a stationary bike or do yoga while watching TV. Walk while taking to friends or family on the phone. Drink a glass of water or a cup of decaf tea. Review how well you met your goals today.

9:00 p.m.

Put the kids to bed, turn down the lights and spend a few moments with your partner. Give each other back rubs, do something special for each other, laugh. Perhaps have a G-Spot snack.

9:20 p.m.

Brush your teeth and hair, floss, wash and exfoliate skin, then use a good night cream that contains a 10% vitamin C solution.

9:35 p.m.

Climb into bed and have sex.

10:30 p.m.

Fall asleep being grateful for all that the day has brought you. Get 7 to 8 hours of restful sleep.

THE AUTHENTIC FOOD
shopping list

A shopping list is the start for building your S-Ex-Y Diet toolkit. Never enter a grocery store without it! Otherwise, you'll impulse buy the Cheetos and forget the broccoli! Make copies of this list and post it on the refrigerator. That way you can jot down needed items and stay organized and focused when you head out the door.

Produce: Fruits & Vegetables

In the Produce Department

- ☐ All colorful, fresh fruits and vegetables
- ☐ Mushrooms
- ☐ Fresh herbs

Down the Aisles

- ☐ Fruits canned in their own juices
- ☐ Bottled 100% orange, grapefruit, tomato, V8 or prune juice
- ☐ Dried fruit
- ☐ Canned tomatoes: paste, stewed, whole
- ☐ Low-fat marinara sauce (such as Francesco Rinaldi ToBe Healthy Sauces)
- ☐ Salsa

In the Refrigerator Case

- ☐ Cartons of 100% orange or grapefruit juice

In the Freezer Case

- ☐ Plain vegetables (not potatoes)
- ☐ Fruit, such as berries, peaches and cherries
- ☐ Concentrated 100% orange juice

Grains & Cereals

In the Bakery

- ☐ 100% whole grains: breads, bagels, English muffins, pita bread and rolls

Down the Aisles

- ☐ Wheat germ
- ☐ Corn or whole-wheat tortillas (especially Mission Life Balance tortillas with DHA)
- ☐ Whole-wheat crackers such as Triscuits
- ☐ Air-popped popcorn
- ☐ Brown rice (instant or regular), brown basmati or texmati rice, Wehani rice, black rice, wild rice
- ☐ Hot cereals such as old-fashioned rolled oats, Kashi, bulgur, quinoa and barley
- ☐ Whole-grain ready-to-eat cereals, such as Shredded Wheat, NutriGrain, Post Whole Wheat Raisin Bran, Grapenuts, low-fat granola, Puffed Kashi
- ☐ Pasta, such as whole wheat or whole-wheat blend noodles
- ☐ Flour, such as whole wheat, rye, oat

In the Freezer Case

- ☐ Whole-grain waffles

Meat, Fish & Legumes

In the Meat Department

- ☐ Extra-lean cuts (no more than 7% fat by weight)
- ☐ Poultry breast without skin
- ☐ All seafood (except tilapia, which has a fat content more like beef than fish)

Down the Aisles

- ☐ Canned tuna, clams or salmon, packed in water (limit intake of tuna to no more than 6 ounces/week)

- [ ] All dried beans and peas, including kidney, black, garbanzo, navy, soybean, lentils, split peas and lima; canned cooked dried beans and peas (beans in "dishes" such as chili or baked beans should be chosen on an individual basis by their fat and sodium content); packaged bean mixes, such as hummus and lentil pilaf (check sodium content)
- [ ] Nut butters, including peanut, almond, soy and cashew
- [ ] Fat-free refried beans

Milk & Other High-Calcium Items

In the Dairy Case

- [ ] 1% or nonfat milk
- [ ] Plain low-fat or nonfat yogurt
- [ ] Nonfat buttermilk
- [ ] DHA-fortified products, such as Horizon Milk with DHA Omega-3 (available in fat free, 2% and whole milk); Horizon Low-fat Chocolate Milk Plus DHA Omega-3; Silk DHA Omega-3 & Calcium; Silk Plus DHA Omega-3 Fortified Soy Beverage
- [ ] Fat-free or low-fat cottage cheese, low-fat cheeses, fresh mozzarella cheese, soy cheese, fat-free or low-fat ricotta cheese, fat-free cream cheese, fat-free sour cream, fat-free half & half, fat-free whipped cream
- [ ] Eggs or egg substitutes
- [ ] Calcium- and vitamin D-fortified orange or grapefruit juice

Down the Aisles

- [ ] Canned fat-free milk

Oils & Fats

Down the Aisles

- [ ] Olive oil, nut oils
- [ ] Fat-free or low-calorie salad dressing
- [ ] Salad spritzers
- [ ] Fat-free or low-calorie mayonnaise. Choose varieties with the omega-3 DHA when possible (such as Pompein OlivExtra Plus)

Sweets & Desserts

Down the Aisles

- [ ] Jam
- [ ] Honey
- [ ] Baby food prunes (as fat replacement in recipes)
- [ ] Cookies made from 100% whole grains

In the Freezer Case

- [ ] Frozen 100% fruit bars and fruit ices
- [ ] Low-fat ice creams and sorbets

Condiments

Down the Aisles

- [ ] Vinegars
- [ ] Mustards
- [ ] Baker's yeast
- [ ] Herbs and spices

HOW **SEXY IS** YOUR MIND?*

Take the quiz and total your score to see how well you are caring for your brain.

A. DIET: 20 Points Out of 60 Possible (33.3% of your total score)

1. How many servings of fatty fish (salmon, tuna, mackerel, trout, whitefish or herring) do you eat in a typical week?

(A) 4 or more servings 7   (B) 2 or 3 5   (C) 1 2   (D) None 0

2. How many times do you consume foods, beverages or supplements fortified with DHA omega-3 in a typical week?

(A) 7 or more times 7   (B) 3–6 times 5   (C) 1–2 times 2   (D) Not at all 0

3. How many servings of colorful fruits and vegetables do you eat in a typical day? (Potatoes and iceberg lettuce do not count.)

(A) 9 or more servings 6   (B) 5–8 servings 4   (C) 2–4 servings 2   (D) 1 or less 0

B. PHYSICAL: 14 Points Out of 60 Possible (23.3% of your total score)

4. Which of the following conditions do you currently have? Select all that apply.

(A) High blood pressure 0   (B) High cholesterol 0   (C) Both -4   (D) Neither -1

5. In a typical week, how many hours do you exercise?

(A) 5 or more hours 4   (B) 3–4 hours 3   (C) 1–2 hours 1   (D) Not at all 0

6. Do you currently smoke?

(A) Yes 0   (B) No 4

7. What is your BMI?

(A) How tall are you? Feet: _____, Inches: _____   (B) How much do you weigh? Pounds: _____

Calculate BMI: Multiply your weight by 705. Divide that number by your height in inches. Divide that number by your height in inches again. That amount equals your current body mass index, or BMI.

(A) < 25 6   (B) 25–29.9 1   (C) ≥30 -2

C. MENTAL: 14 Points Out of 60 Possible (23.3% of your total score)

8. How happy would you say you currently are?

(A) Very happy   3   (B) Pretty happy   2   (C) Not too happy   1   (D) I'm sad   0

9. Have any of your blood relatives had Alzheimer's disease/dementia?

(A) Yes   0   (B) No   2

10. How many minutes do you spend playing games or learning a new skill in a typical day? (Examples: playing board games/Scrabble/cards, playing computer games, doing jigsaw or crossword puzzles, learning a new language)

(A) 31 or more   (B) 11–30 minutes   4   (C) 1–10 minutes   2   (D) Not at all   0
minutes   5

11. How many minutes do you spend reading for personal interest in a typical day? (Examples: reading a magazine/book/newspaper)

(A) 46 or more   (B) 16–45 minutes   3   (C) 5–15 minutes   2   (D) Not at all   0
minutes   4

D. SOCIAL: 12 Points Out of 60 Possible (20% of your total score)

12. How many hours do you volunteer or help out a friend in a typical month?

(A) 6 or more hours   3   (B) 3–5 hours   2   (C) 1–2 hours   1   (D) Not at all   0

13. How often do you get the social and emotional support you need?

(A) Always   9   (B) Usually   7   (C) Sometimes   5   (D) Rarely   2   (E) Never   0

Tally Your Score:

Points   What This Means

31–60   You have a sexy mind. You embody the four dimensions of brain health. You know what it takes to keep your mind in tip-top shape. Don't slow down. Keep up the good work. If your score is closer to 31 than to 60, note where you need improvement and get on with it!

11–30   You are a sexy mind apprentice. You are obviously conscientious about good health. Learn what you can do to take it to the next level, which is sure to up your sexy quotient.

0–10   You are a sexy mind beginner. There's a lot you need to do ASAP to improve the overall health of your brain. Aim to increase your score by 10 points in the next month. Then keep going from there.

*Excerpted with permission from: The *life's*DHA Brain Health Quiz, a part of the Beautiful Minds Campaign (www.beautiful-minds.com), a partnership between Martek Biosciences and the National Center for Creative Aging to help raise awareness of the actions people can take to better maintain brain health.

A WEEK'S WORTH OF
sexy menus

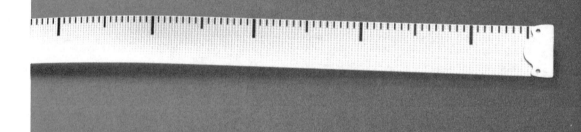

Need a sexy game plan? Here's a week's worth of delicious, turn-me-on meals and snacks, guaranteed to rev up your motor, improve your mood, boost energy, help you think a little faster, and even drop a pound or two. Each day's menu supplies all your needs for vitamins, minerals, fiber and other feel-good, look-great nutrients—all for less than 2,000 calories. If you want to lose weight faster, drop one or two of the snacks. The recipes can be found starting on page 210.

1 serving Sauced and Bedded Egg Florentine *(from Recipe section)*

1 cup Tropicana orange juice

Tea

Midmorning Snack

1 2" oatmeal-raisin cookie

1 cup soymilk w/DHA

Lunch

Peanut Butter Candy Sandwich: Blend 2 tablespoons peanut butter, 2 tablespoons toasted wheat germ and 1 tablespoon honey. Spread on 2 slices 100% whole-grain bread.

1 cup sliced sweet red pepper

1 cup nonfat milk, warmed and sprinkled with nutmeg

Midafternoon Snack

1 ounce almonds *(approximately 12)*

3 graham crackers

Water

Dinner

4 ounces roast chicken breast *(Save extra chicken for salad later in the week.)*

1 cup steamed Brussels sprouts

1 cup mashed potatoes made with 1% low-fat milk

Sparkling water with lime juice

Glazed Carrots: 2 carrots, peeled and sliced into ¼" diagonals, cooked in 1 teaspoon olive oil and ¼ cup orange juice until tender. In a small bowl, mix until smooth ½ teaspoon cornstarch, ¼ teaspoon ground ginger, pinch of nutmeg and 3 tablespoons water. Add ginger mixture to carrots and stir over medium heat until sauce thickens. Sprinkle with 2 teaspoons chopped chives and a pinch of red pepper flakes (optional).

Late-Night Snack

1 cup frozen blueberries

Nutritional Analysis: 1,999 calories, 30% fat (66.6 g; 13.6 g saturated), 50% carbs (250 g), 20% protein (100 g), 34 g fiber, 1,587 mg sodium

DAY 2

Breakfast

½ cup oatmeal cooked in ½ cup 1% low-fat milk, topped with 1 teaspoon chopped walnuts and 2 teaspoons maple syrup

1 cup melon with ½ cup plain, nonfat yogurt

Midmorning Snack

Fruity Burrito: Spread 2 tablespoons fat-free cream cheese and 2 teaspoons all-fruit jam on a heated 8" Life Balance flour tortilla. Fill with ⅓ cup fresh fruit such as peach slices and strawberries, and roll into a burrito.

Sparkling water with lemon

Lunch

1 **serving** Spicy Thai 'em Up Sweet Potato Soup *(from Recipe section)*

1 slice whole-wheat bread

½ mango, peeled, seeded and sliced

Midafternoon Snack

3 fat-free whole-wheat crackers, topped with 2 teaspoons peanut butter and 1 teaspoon jam

1 cup baby carrots

Water

Dinner

Sushi Salmon: Blend 1 tablespoon light soy sauce, ¼ teaspoon wasabi powder and ½ teaspoon minced fresh ginger in a small bowl. Rub on a 4-ounce salmon fillet. Broil for 5 to 10 minutes (depending on thickness of fish, or until center is no longer translucent).

½ 6-ounce baked garnet sweet potato

1 cup steamed broccoli

½ cup cooked brown rice

Late-Night Snack

1 baked apple stuffed with 1 tablespoon chopped walnuts, ½ teaspoon ground cinnamon and 2 teaspoons brown sugar

Nutrition Analysis: 1,988 calories, 21% fat (46 g; 10 g saturated), 63% carbs (313 g), 16% protein (79.6 g), 41 g fiber, 2,273 mg sodium

DAY 3

Breakfast

1 2-ounce, low-fat bran muffin topped with 1 tablespoon cashew, almond or peanut butter

Fruit Salad: ½ cup pineapple chunks (fresh or canned in their own juice) and 1 kiwi fruit, peeled and sliced. *(optional: sprinkle with ½ teaspoon crystalized ginger)*

1 cup soymilk w/DHA

Midmorning Snack

⅔ cup plain, nonfat yogurt mixed with 2 tablespoons pomegranate seeds and 1 teaspoon honey

Lunch

1 serving Zesty Shrimp and Spinach Salad *(from Recipe section)*

1 slice French bread

Midafternoon snack

3 whole-wheat crackers, topped with 2 teaspoons fat-free cream cheese, 1 slice Granny Smith apple, and 1 bread and butter pickle slice

Water

Dinner

3 ounces roasted pork loin

1 cup A Sexy Little Roast Vegetable Number *(from Recipe section)*

Tossed salad made with 3 cups Tender Ruby Red lettuce, 1 slice red onion, 1 chopped tomato and 2 tablespoons low-fat dressing

1 whole-wheat dinner roll with 2 teaspoons butter

½ whole-wheat bagel, toasted and topped with 2 teaspoons apricot jam

Decaf Earl Grey tea *(optional: sweetened with Splenda)*

Nutrition Analysis: 1,946 calories, 33% fat (71 g; 16.8 g saturated), 46% carbs (224 g), 21% protein (102 g), 34 g fiber, 2,391 mg sodium

DAY 4

Breakfast

Berry Parfait: Layer the following in a tall glass: 1 cup plain, nonfat yogurt; ⅓ cup low-fat granola; and 1 ¼ cups berries (fresh or thawed and drained frozen).

1 cup calcium- and vitamin D-fortified orange juice

Green tea *(optional)*

Midmorning Snack

¼ cup dried figs and 1 ounce almonds *(approximately 12)*

Water

Lunch

Bagel Melt: ½ 5-ounce 100% whole-wheat bagel. Top with 3 tomato slices, 1 slice red onion and 1 ounce low-fat cheddar cheese. Broil until cheese bubbles.

Coleslaw: 1 cup shredded cabbage mixed with 1 tablespoon low-fat dressing.

Midafternoon Snack

2 cups watermelon cubes

1 Orange-Scented Swiss Kiss *(from Recipe section)*

Dinner

Broiled Halibut with Corn Salsa: 5 ounces halibut steak, brushed with lemon juice and black pepper. Place steak on broiler pan and broil, 4 inches below heating element, for 10 minutes per inch of thickness or until fish flakes easily. Top with ½ cup corn salsa (commercial brand or homemade from lime juice, corn, diced red onion, cilantro, red pepper and jalapeño pepper).

½ cup cooked brown rice mixed with fresh herbs and ¼ cup green peas

15 asparagus spears lightly sautéed with 1 minced clove garlic in nonstick frying pan coated with cooking spray

1 cup canned mandarin oranges, drained and topped with 2 table-spoons pomegranate seeds and 1 teaspoon crystalized ginger

Decaffeinated tea *(optional: sweetened with sugar substitute)*

Late-Night Snack

2 cups air-popped popcorn

Nutrition Analysis: 1,948 calories, 17% fat (37 g; 8.3 g saturated), 65% carbs (317 g), 18% protein (88 g), 479 g fiber, 1,017 mg sodium

DAY 5

Breakfast

1 serving Apple-of-My-Eye Popover Pancake *(from Recipe section)*

6 ounces apricot nectar

Midmorning Snack

2 fresh figs

1 ounce low-fat cheese

Green tea

Lunch

Lox & Bagel: **Toast one half of a 4-ounce whole-grain bagel and top with 2 tablespoons fat-free cream cheese, 2 ounces smoked salmon, 1 red onion slice, ¼ cup alfalfa sprouts and 4 slices tomato.**

½ cup watermelon chunks

Water

Midafternoon Snack

PB & F Roll-Up: **Spread 1 tablespoon nut butter on a tortilla. Top with ⅓ cup fresh fruit and roll into a burrito.**

Water

Dinner

1 slice Passionate Peppered Pizza *(from Recipe section)*

Tall glass of sparkling water mixed with ½ cup orange juice

Wild Baby Greens with Pears: 3 cups wild baby greens (or any leaf lettuce), 2 tablespoons dried figs, ½ large red pear, sliced, fresh herbs and 3 tablespoons low-calorie dressing, such as Newman's Own Sesame Ginger Dressing.

Late-Night Snack

½ cup sorbet topped with ⅔ cup berries

Nutrition Analysis: 1,918 calories, 17% fat (36 g; 9 g saturated), 69% carbs (331 g), 14% protein (67 g), 44 g fiber, 2,560 mg sodium

DAY 6

Breakfast

1 serving Seriously Sensuous Honeyed Fig Oatmeal *(from Recipe section)*

6 ounces calcium- and vitamin D-fortified orange juice

Green tea *(optional)*

Midmorning Snack

1 nonfat latte

1 fig bar cookie

Lunch

All-Veggie Spaghetti: Top 2 cups cooked spaghetti squash with ½ cup commercial spaghetti sauce and 2 tablespoon low-fat Parmesan cheese.

1 serving Fall Romance Salad *(from Recipe section)*

Sparkling water with lemon

Midafternoon Snack

½ cup plain, nonfat yogurt, topped with 1 tablespoon honey and 2 tablespoons dried fruit

Water

Dinner

1 serving Some Like it Hot Orange-Chipotle Chicken *(from Recipe section)*

½ cup smashed sweet potatoes *(bake or microwave garnet sweet potatoes until soft, spoon out insides, mix with a little honey, salt and pepper)*

⅔ cup fresh or frozen and steamed green beans

Late-Night Snack

1 slice Berry Quickie Ice Cream Pie *(from Recipe section)*

Decaf tea

Nutrition Analysis: 1,951 calories, 25% fat (54 g; 8.7 g saturated), 59% carbs (288 g), 16% protein (78 g), 36 g fiber, 1,494 mg sodium

DAY 7

Breakfast

1 slice 100% whole-wheat toast, topped with 1 tablespoon peanut butter and ¼ cup pineapple chunks

Coffee or tea with ⅓ cup low-fat 1% milk

Midmorning Snack

1 small (2 ounce) low-fat bran muffin topped with 2 tablespoons apple butter

1 cup soymilk w/DHA

Water

Lunch

On-the-Go Deli Lunch:

1 turkey breast sandwich on 100% whole-wheat bread with mustard and lettuce *(3 ounces turkey)*

1 cup sliced cucumbers marinated in vinegar and spices

1 large apple

Diet soda or sparkling water

Midafternoon Snack

Guacamole and Chips: Blend ¼ cup avocado cubes, ¼ cup chopped tomato, 1 tablespoon canned chili pepper, 2 table-spoons diced cilantro and salt/pepper to taste. Dip 16 baked tortilla chips and ½ cup jicama strips in the dip.

Dinner

1 serving Kissed by an Italian Penne (with the Touch of an Eggplant and Zucchini) *(from Recipe section)*

1 cup sautéed spinach *(lightly sautéed in olive oil and minced garlic)*

1 glass red wine *(optional)*

Late-Night Snack

1 slice Is-That-a-Carrot-in-Your-Pocket-or-Are-You-Just-Glad-to-See-Me Cake *(from Recipe section)*

Nutrition Analysis: 1,940 calories, 25% fat (54 g; 10 g saturated), 54% carbs (262 g), 17% protein (82.5 g), 4% alcohol, 41 g fiber, 2,394 mg sodium

get-in-the-mood
RECIPES

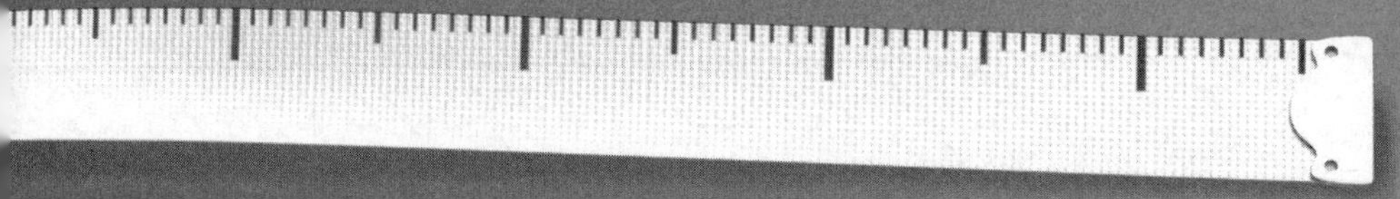

Apple-of-My-Eye Popover Pancake

Ingredients

1 tablespoon butter

2 pounds apples (Gala, Fuji or golden delicious), peeled, seeded and cut into ¼" wedges

½ cup dried tart cherries

3 tablespoons sugar

4 tablespoons Splenda

¼ cup apple juice concentrate

½ teaspoon almond extract

⅓ cup whole-wheat flour

⅓ cup unbleached white flour

¼ teaspoon salt

1 cup low-fat milk or soymilk

¾ cup liquid egg substitute

1 tablespoon light olive oil or canola oil

1 teaspoon sesame seeds

2 cups nonfat, plain yogurt

Directions

Heat oven to 420°F.

1 Melt butter in a nonstick frying pan over medium-high heat. Add apples, cherries, 2 tablespoons sugar and 2 tablespoons Splenda, and cook until apples are light golden and soft, approximately 15 minutes. Add apple juice concentrate and extract, and cook until liquid is thick, approximately 3 minutes. Remove from heat.

2 In a medium bowl, place flours, salt and the rest of the sugar and Splenda. Blend thoroughly.

3 In a small bowl, whip milk and egg substitute. Add to flour mixture and stir until thoroughly blended.

4 Heat a 12" cast-iron frying pan, add oil to coat the entire bottom of pan. Remove from heat, pour in batter, and bake until golden and fluffy, approximately 15 minutes. Remove from oven.

5 Place apple mixture in pancake and spread to cover bottom. Sprinkle with sesame seeds, cut into 6 wedges. Serve topped with ⅓ cup yogurt. Makes 6 servings.

Nutrition Analysis: 326 calories, 18% fat (6.5 g; 2.3 g saturated), 67% carbs (54.6 g), 15% protein (12.3 g), 5 g fiber, 252 mg sodium

Sauced and Bedded Egg Florentine

Directions

1 Fill a large skillet with 2–3 inches of water. Add vinegar and bring to a simmer over medium-high heat.

2 While water is coming to a boil, make hollandaise sauce: Combine egg yolk, milk, flour, mustard, Tabasco, salt and pepper in a small saucepan. Whisk until thoroughly blended. Heat over medium heat until sauce simmers and thickens slightly. Remove from heat and add lemon juice. Set aside. Add an additional tablespoon of milk if sauce is too thick.

3 While water is coming to a boil, toast muffins. Set aside. Place spinach in a bowl, cover and microwave for 1 minute or until leaves are wilted. Drain extra fluid.

4 Gently crack eggs, one at a time, into small bowls or ramekins. Gently slide each egg, one at a time, into the simmering water. Simmer for 4 to 5 minutes or until whites are cooked and yolk is the desired consistency. Use a slotted spoon to remove each egg.

5 Divide spinach evenly between the 4 toasted muffin halves, place an egg on top of the spinach and spoon sauce over the top. Makes 4 servings.

Ingredients

1 tablespoon white vinegar

1 egg yolk

⅔ cup fat-free evaporated milk

2 teaspoons unbleached flour

¼ teaspoon Dijon mustard

Tabasco sauce

Salt and pepper to taste

2 tablespoons lemon juice

2 100% whole-grain English muffins, split

2 cups baby spinach

4 whole eggs

Nutrition Analysis per serving: 191 calories, 32% fat (6.8 g; 2 g saturated), 40% carbs (19 g), 28% protein (13.4 g), 2.6 g fiber, 310 mg sodium

Seriously Sensuous Honeyed Fig Oatmeal

Ingredients

1 ¼ cups 1% low-fat milk or plain soymilk with DHA

1 cup old-fashioned oats

2 tablespoons toasted wheat germ

1 teaspoon vanilla

¼ cup water

4 dried figs, chopped

2 tablespoons chopped pecans

¼ teaspoon cardamom

1 tablespoon honey

½ teaspoon vanilla

¼ cup fat-free half & half

Directions

1 Bring milk to a gentle boil, add oats and wheat germ. Stir and cover. Reduce heat and simmer until almost done. Stir in vanilla, cover, then set aside to soak up remaining liquid.

2 In a saucepan over medium-high heat, add ¼ cup water, figs, pecans, cardamom, honey and vanilla. Simmer until liquid forms a glaze. Remove from heat.

3 Divide and place oatmeal into two bowls. Top with fig mixture and pour half & half around the edges. Makes 2 servings.

Nutrition Analysis per serving: 432 calories, 23% fat (11 g; 1 g saturated), 65% carbs (70 g), 12% protein (13 g), 9 g fiber, 81 mg sodium

Spicy Thai 'em Up Sweet Potato Soup

Directions

1 In a large saucepan, heat oil over medium heat. Add onion and sauté, stirring frequently, for 4 minutes. Add sweet potato, turn up heat to medium-high and sauté, stirring frequently, for 10 minutes. Add garlic, ginger, chutney, peanut butter and curry paste, and stir to thoroughly coat sweet potatoes. Add vermouth, stir and simmer until liquid is slightly reduced, approximately 5 minutes. Add broth and potato, bring to boil, reduce heat and simmer uncovered until potatoes begin to break apart, approximately 30 minutes. Add lime juice and zest.

2 Transfer soup to food processor or blender and purée. Return to saucepan, add coconut milk, evaporated milk and honey. Simmer uncovered for 5 minutes. Salt and pepper to taste. Pour into soup bowls and garnish with peanuts and cilantro. Makes 6 servings *(approximately 2 cups each)*.

Ingredients

1 tablespoon olive oil

1 cup chopped yellow onion

10 cups sweet potato (peeled and cubed, approximately 3½–4 pounds of whole potato)

2 minced garlic cloves

1 tablespoon minced fresh ginger root

⅓ cup spicy mango chutney

3 tablespoons creamy peanut butter

2 tablespoons red curry paste

⅓ cup vermouth

6 cups chicken broth

1 8-ounce baker potato, peeled and cubed

Juice and zest from 1 lime

½ cup lite coconut milk

½ cup fat-free evaporated milk

1 tablespoon honey

Salt and pepper to taste

2 tablespoons finely chopped peanuts

2 tablespoons chopped cilantro

Nutrition Analysis: 464 calories, 20% fat (10 g; 2.6 g saturated), 67% carbs (77g), 13% protein (15.1 g), 9 g fiber, 863 mg sodium

Zesty Shrimp and Spinach Salad

Ingredients

¼ cup extra-virgin olive oil

¼ cup lemon juice

1 tablespoon finely grated lemon zest

1 minced garlic clove

1 teaspoon Dijon mustard

1 teaspoon Splenda

Salt and pepper

1 cup uncooked whole-grain rotini pasta

1 peeled, seeded and cubed avocado

1 generous cup halved cherry tomatoes

¼ cup chopped red onion

3 tablespoons chopped fresh cilantro

1 pound precooked, peeled, deveined large shrimp

4 cups baby spinach

Directions

1 In a small bowl, combine oil, lemon juice, lemon zest, garlic, mustard, Splenda and salt and pepper *(to taste)*. Set aside.

2 Bring 6 cups water to a boil, add pasta and cook according to directions on package, or until al dente. Drain and rinse.

3 While pasta is cooking, combine avocado, tomatoes, onion, cilantro and shrimp. Add pasta and toss. Add dressing and toss.

4 Place 1 cup baby spinach on each of 4 plates. Top with shrimp-pasta mixture. Makes 4 servings.

Nutrition Analysis per serving: 436 calories, 45% fat (21.8 g; 3.6 g saturated), 28% carbs (30.5 g), 27% protein (29.4 g), 7.1 g fiber, 314 mg sodium

A Toss in the Hay with Corn, Sweet Potatoes and Black Beans

Directions

Heat oven to 425°F. Coat cookie sheet with cooking spray.

1 Place sweet potatoes on cookie sheet, sprinkle lightly with salt and pepper and spray with cooking spray. Roast for 10 minutes or until slightly cooked, but still firm. Remove from oven and cool.

2 In a large bowl, combine corn, tomatoes, peppers, onion and beans. Add cooled sweet potatoes. Set aside.

3 In a small bowl, blend vinegar, oil, mustard, and salt and pepper to taste. Drizzle over sweet potato mixture and toss to evenly coat.

4 Arrange 1 cup of greens on each of 4 plates. Top with sweet potato mixture. Makes 4 servings.

Ingredients

Cooking spray

2 cups peeled and cubed sweet potatoes (yams)

Salt and pepper

2 cups fresh or frozen corn kernels

1 cup halved cherry tomatoes

1 ¼ cups diced red bell pepper

½ cup thinly sliced and cut red onion

1 cup canned black beans, drained and rinsed

3 tablespoons balsamic vinegar

3 tablespoons extra virgin olive oil

1 tablespoon Dijon mustard

4 cups wild greens or baby spinach

Nutrition Analysis per serving: 315 calories, 32% fat (11.2 g; 1.7 g saturated), 56% carbs (44 g), 12% protein (9.5 g), 10 g fiber, 86 mg sodium

215

Red Hot Mama Beet Salad

Ingredients

Cooking spray

12 small-sized beets or
6 medium-sized beets, with stems
and tails removed

Salt and pepper to taste

1 ½ cups orange juice

1 tablespoon lemon juice

1 tablespoon cooking sherry

2 tablespoons extra virgin olive oil

½ cup chopped pecans

1 tablespoon maple syrup

4 cups lettuce (Tender Ruby Reds
go well with this salad)

¼ cup crumbled blue cheese

Directions

Heat oven to 425°F. Coat cookie sheet with cooking spray.

1 Spread beets (whole if small or cut in half if medium) on cookie sheet, sprinkle with salt and pepper, coat with cooking spray and roast for 40 minutes, or until firm, but slightly tender when pierced with a fork. Turn once or twice during roasting. Remove from oven to cool. Peel and cut into bite-sized chunks.

2 While beets are roasting, place orange juice in a medium saucepan and simmer until reduced to ⅓ cup and mixture has a slight syrupy consistency. Add lemon juice, sherry and salt and return to simmer for 3 minutes. Remove from heat, cool slightly and add oil. Adjust seasonings.

3 In a small bowl, toss pecans with maple syrup, transfer to tinfoil or cookie sheet coated with cooking spray and roast for 5 minutes at 425°F. Remove from oven and cool slightly.

4 Drizzle 1 tablespoon of dressing over beets and toss. Add the rest of the dressing to the lettuce and toss until thoroughly coated. Transfer lettuce to each of 4 plates, top with beets, 1 tablespoon each blue cheese and pecans. Makes 4 servings.

Nutrition Analysis per serving: 340 calories, 50% fat (18.9 g; 3.4 g saturated), 41% carbs (35 g), 9% protein (7.7 g), 7 g fiber, 251 mg sodium

My Little Chickadee Stew

Directions

1 In a large saucepan over medium-high heat, place oil, onions, carrots and celery. Stir until tender, approximately 5 minutes. Add garlic and sweet potato and continue to sauté for another 2 minutes. Add the next 8 ingredients *(through the chicken)*. Return to simmer and cook, uncovered, until potatoes are firm but tender, approximately 15 minutes. Adjust seasoning.

2 Place 1 cup brown rice in each bowl, top with 2 cups of stew, a sprinkle of cilantro and 2 tablespoons sour cream.
Makes 4 generous servings.

Ingredients

1 tablespoon olive oil

2 cups diced yellow onion

2 cups diced carrots

½ cup diced celery

3 minced garlic cloves

1 8-ounce garnet sweet potato, peeled and cubed (approx. 1 ¾ cups)

1 4-ounce can diced green chilies

2 ½ teaspoons ground cumin

1 teaspoon turmeric

1 ½ teaspoons chili powder

1 14-ounce can low-sodium chicken broth

1 15-ounce can chickpeas, drained and rinsed

1 28-ounce can low-sodium diced tomatoes

8 ounces cooked and diced skinless chicken breast

Salt and pepper to taste

4 cups cooked brown rice

½ cup chopped cilantro

½ cup fat-free sour cream

Nutrition Analysis per serving: 423 calories, 18% fat (8.5 g; 1.5 g saturated), 51% carbs (54 g), 31% protein (33 g), 12 g fiber, 520 mg sodium

Loving Spoonfuls of Carrot-Ginger Soup

Ingredients

1 tablespoon olive oil

2 cups diced yellow onion

1 pound carrots, peeled and cut into thin rounds, plus 1 carrot peeled and diced

1 12-ounce russet potato, peeled and chopped

3 minced garlic cloves

2 tablespoons grated, fresh ginger root

5 cups low-sodium chicken broth

2 tablespoons honey

½ cup fat-free half & half

⅛ teaspoon curry powder

Salt and white pepper to taste

¼ cup finely chopped parsley

Directions

1 In a large saucepan, heat oil over medium-high heat. Add onions and stir for 5 minutes, or until slightly transparent. Add carrots and potato. Continue to stir until carrots are heated through and slightly tender. Add garlic and ginger, and cook for another 3 minutes. Add broth, return to simmer, and cook for 20 minutes, uncovered, or until vegetables are very tender.

2 Transfer mixture to blender or food processor and purée in batches until smooth.

3 Return to saucepan, add diced carrots and cook for 7 minutes, or until carrots are soft. Add honey, half & half, curry, and salt and pepper (*if desired*). Garnish each bowl with parsley.
Makes 4 servings.

Nutrition Analysis: 290 calories, 17% fat (5.5 g; 1 g saturated), 68% carbs (49 g), 15% protein (11 g), 7 g fiber, 155 mg sodium

Fall Romance Salad

Directions

1 Dressing: In a medium, nonstick saucepan, bring juice to a gentle boil and simmer until reduced to ¾ cup, approximately 20 minutes. Set aside to cool. While still warm, add thyme. When cool, add vinegar, oil, pepper and salt.

2 Salad: Place lettuce in a large bowl. Top with onion, parsley, walnuts, orange pieces and, finally, pomegranate seeds. When ready to serve, gently and thoroughly toss with dressing.
Makes 8 servings.

Ingredients

Dressing:
2 ⅓ cups unsweetened pomegranate juice

2 teaspoons fresh thyme leaves

4 tablespoons red wine vinegar (preferably one infused with pomegranate)

3 tablespoons extra virgin olive oil

½ teaspoon fresh-ground pepper

Salt to taste

Salad:
20 ounces baby greens, such as Fresh Express Tender Ruby Reds

⅓ cup thinly sliced red onion

¼ cup chopped flat-leaf parsley

2 cups toasted walnut pieces

5 tangerines or small mandarin oranges, peeled, sectioned, the pith removed and cut in half

1 ½ cups pomegranate seeds

Nutrition Analysis per serving: 332 calories, 61% fat (22 g; 2 g saturated), 32% carbs (27 g), 7% protein (5.8 g), 3.8 g fiber, 13 mg sodium

Wham Bam Thank You Ma'am Calzone

Ingredients

Cooking spray

1 refrigerated pizza crust

1 tablespoon olive oil

1 medium yellow onion, peeled and chopped

3 minced garlic cloves

1 bag 16-ounce frozen Asparagus Stir Fry (or your favorite frozen vegetables)

6 ounces frozen chopped spinach, thawed and drained

½ cup chopped fresh basil (optional)

1 tablespoon Italian herbs

1 ¼ cups shredded low-fat mozzarella

4 tablespoons grated low-fat Parmesan

1 whipped egg white

1 cup hot low-sodium spaghetti sauce

Directions

Heat oven to 425°F. Coat cookie sheet with cooking spray.

1 Take pizza-crust dough out of the packaging. Spread into a rectangle and cut into halves. Place on cookie sheet. Set aside.

2 Heat oil in a large, nonstick pan over medium-high heat. Add onions and sauté until translucent, approximately 5 minutes. Add garlic, vegetables and herbs. Toss and cook until hot.

3 Place half of the vegetable mixture on each of the 2 crust halves. Top each with half the cheeses. Bring sides of crust together and pinch to seal. Brush with egg white and cut 3 slits into tops to allow steam to escape. Place in oven and bake until golden, about 15 minutes. Allow to cool for 5 minutes.

4 Cut each calzone in half. Place on plates and top with spaghetti sauce.
Makes 4 servings.

Nutrition Analysis per serving: 478 calories, 33% fat (17 g; 5.6 g saturated), 49% carbs (59 g), 18% protein (21.5 g), 5 g fiber, 799 mg sodium

Nuts About You Curried Chicken Bowl

This tasty salad can top lettuce greens for a meal salad or works as a great sandwich mix. Just top with lots of lettuce and use whole-grain bread.

Directions

In a medium bowl, combine ingredients from mayonnaise to nuts until thoroughly blended. Add chicken, toss to blend, and season with salt and pepper to taste. Makes 4 servings.

Ingredients

½ cup low-fat mayonnaise

2 teaspoons curry powder

1 teaspoon turmeric powder

1 cup peeled and diced Granny Smith apple

⅓ cup finely diced red bell pepper

⅓ cup dried tart cherries

⅓ cup chopped nuts (peanuts are particularly good, but any nut will do)

2 cups diced cooked skinless chicken breast

Salt and pepper to taste

Nutrition Analysis per serving: 291 calories, 41% fat (13 g; 2.4 g saturated), 31% carbs (22.6 g), 28% protein (20.4 g), 2.5 g fiber, 75 mg sodium

Ya' Wanna Pizza Me!

Ingredients

1 whole-wheat premade pizza crust, such as Boboli

6 ounces shredded low-fat, low-sodium cheese

1 15-ounce can black beans, drained and rinsed thoroughly

1 cup frozen corn, thawed

1 4-ounce can diced green chilies, drained

⅓ cup diced red onion

1 tablespoon olive oil

Salt to taste

3 large tomatoes, sliced

Directions

Preheat oven to 425°F.

1 Sprinkle pizza crust with 4 ounces of the cheese. Place on baking sheet or pizza pan and set aside.

2 In a medium bowl, mix beans, corn, chilies, onion, oil and salt to taste. Spread mixture evenly over crust and sprinkle with remaining 2 ounces of cheese. Bake for 15 minutes, or until bottom of crust is brown and cheese has thoroughly melted.

3 Cut into quarters or eighths and top with slices of tomato.

Makes 4 servings.

Nutrition Analysis per serving: 460 calories, 21% fat (10.7 g; 4 g saturated), 56% carbs (64 g), 23% protein (26.5 g), 14 g fiber, 703 mg sodium

Lay It on Me Frittata

Directions

1 Spray a 10" nonstick, oven-safe skillet with cooking spray and heat over medium heat. Add onion, cook, stirring often, until transparent, approximately 3–5 minutes. Add garlic and spinach and heat through. Add tomatoes, mint and basil. Heat through until any excess liquid has evaporated. Remove from heat.

2 In a medium bowl, whisk egg substitute with salt, pepper and red pepper flakes. Add spinach mixture. Stir to combine.

3 Whip out skillet and re-spray with cooking spray. Place over medium-low heat, add frittata mixture and cook, without stirring, until bottom is light golden, approximately 5 minutes. As the mixture cooks, lift the edges and tilt the pan so uncooked egg flows to the edges. Sprinkle with cheese.

4 Place skillet under broiler about 4 inches from the element, and cook until frittata is set and top is golden, approximately 2 to 4 minutes. Remove, loosen edges and slide frittata onto a plate or cutting board. Cut into 4 wedges.

Ingredients

Cooking spray

1 medium onion, peeled and chopped (approximately 1 ⅓ cups)

2 minced garlic cloves

1 box frozen chopped spinach, thawed and drained

1 cup cherry tomatoes, halved

¼ cup chopped fresh mint leaves

⅓ cup chopped fresh basil leaves

2 cups liquid egg substitute

Salt and pepper to taste

Pinch of red pepper flakes

½ cup grated low-fat sharp cheddar cheese

Nutrition Analysis per wedge: 194 calories, 27% fat (5.8 g; 1.7 g saturated), 27% carbs (13.1 g), 46% protein (22 g), 4 g fiber, 292 mg sodium

A Sexy Little Roast Vegetable Number

Ingredients

4 cups cauliflower florets

3 cups peeled, seeded and cubed (1" square) butternut squash

3 cups carrots, peeled, halved lengthwise, then halved lengthwise again and cut into 2"-long strips

1 pound Brussels sprouts, trimmed and halved

3 tablespoons olive oil

Salt and pepper

⅓ cup chopped pecans

⅓ cup low-fat, grated Parmesan cheese

⅓ cup finely chopped fresh parsley

1 ½ tablespoons lemon juice

1 tablespoon finely grated lemon peel

2 minced garlic cloves

¼ teaspoon red pepper flakes

Directions

Heat oven to 425°F.

1 In a large bowl, toss cauliflower, squash, carrots, Brussels sprouts, oil, salt and pepper *(to taste)*. Place vegetables on a cookie sheet and roast until firm, but cooked, approximately 30 minutes. Remove and place on platter.

2 While vegetables are roasting, combine the remaining ingredients in a small bowl and toss to blend. Place on top of roasted vegetables just before serving.

Makes 6 servings.

Nutrition Analysis per serving: 232 calories, 46% fat (11.8 g; 1 g saturated), 44% carbs (25 g), 10% protein (5.8 g), 9 g fiber, 142 mg sodium

Passionate Peppered Pizza

Directions

Heat oven to 425°F. Coat cookie sheet with cooking spray.

1 Wrap garlic in tinfoil, spray with cooking spray and seal. Place pepper, eggplant and zucchini on coated cookie sheet. Place garlic and vegetables in the oven and roast for 20 minutes or until tender, turning once or twice. Remove and set aside.

2 Remove garlic from skins and spread evenly on top of the pizza crust. Top with spaghetti sauce, spreading evenly over garlic and crust. Sprinkle with cheese and top with roasted vegetables. Bake for 12 minutes or until cheese begins to bubble and pizza is hot.
Makes 6 slices.

Ingredients

Cooking spray

5 whole garlic cloves in skins

1 red bell pepper, seeded, stemmed and cut into thin strips

2 cups peeled and cubed eggplant

1 zucchini, cut into thin rounds

1 premade commercial whole-wheat pizza crust (such as Boboli)

1 cup bottled spaghetti sauce

4 ounces grated Italian cheese (combination of low-fat mozzarella and Parmesan)

Nutrition Analysis per slice: 247 calories, 28% fat (7.7 g; 2 g saturated), 56% carbs (35 g), 16% protein (10 g), 6 g fiber, 615 mg sodium

Creamy, Sagey Butternutty Risotto

Ingredients

6+ cups chicken broth

1 tablespoon olive oil

1 medium yellow onion, diced

15 large fresh sage leaves, diced

1 medium butternut squash, peeled, seeded and cut into ½" squares

⅔ cup vermouth

1 ½ cups Arborio rice

Parmesan cheese (optional)

Directions

1 Pour broth into a medium saucepan, heat to simmer, reduce heat and keep warm.

2 Heat oil in large, nonstick frying pan. Add onion and stir over medium heat until translucent. Add sage and stir to thoroughly mix. Add squash and cook for 4 minutes, stirring to coat. Add vermouth and 1 cup of the stock. Bring to a boil, reduce heat, cover and simmer until squash is tender, approximately 30 minutes. Uncover and let extra liquid cook off.

3 Add rice to squash, stir until thoroughly mixed. Add ½ cup of warm broth and stir frequently until rice absorbs the liquid. Continue to add broth ½ cup at a time while stirring, until the rice is creamy and soft, but still al dente and the squash blends into the broth, approximately 30 minutes.

4 Remove from heat, add Parmesan *(if desired)*. Serve immediately.
Makes 6 generous servings.

Nutrition Analysis: 418 calories, 16% fat (7.4 g;1 g saturated), 66% carbs (69 g), 18% protein (9 g), 16 g fiber, 930 mg sodium

Mango Salsa Dancing Caribbean Chicken

Directions

Heat oven to 425°F. Coat a cookie sheet with cooking spray.

1 Salsa: Combine all ingredients in a small bowl. Set aside for flavors to blend.

2 Chicken: Evenly sprinkle chicken breast halves with seasoning mix. Place on coated cookie sheet and bake until done, approximately 20 minutes. (*Do not overcook, or chicken will be dry.*)

3 Place a chicken breast on each plate, pile with salsa, garnish with a lime wedge and cilantro sprig. Makes 4 servings.

Ingredients

Salsa:
1 mango, peeled, seeded and diced (approximately 1 ½ cups)

3 tablespoons diced red onion

3 tablespoons diced red bell pepper

2 tablespoons minced fresh cilantro

2 tablespoons canned diced green chilies

2 tablespoons fresh lime juice

Chicken:
Cooking spray

4 4-ounce skinless, boneless chicken breast halves

3 tablespoons no-salt Caribbean citrus seasoning mix

Lime wedges

Cilantro sprigs

Nutrition Analysis per serving: 164 calories, 9% fat (1.6 g; <1 g saturated), 26% carbs (10.7 g), 65% protein (26.7 g), 1.3 g fiber, 75 mg sodium

Some Like it Hot Orange-Chipotle Chicken

DINNERS

Ingredients

2 teaspoons minced
chipotle chilies in adobo sauce

¾ cup orange marmalade

2 tablespoons minced red onion

2 tablespoons minced
fresh cilantro

Cooking spray

Salt and pepper

4 4-ounce skinless, boneless
chicken breast halves

2½ cups cooked brown rice

Directions

1 In a small bowl, mix first 4 ingredients until thoroughly blended. Set aside for flavors to blend.

2 Spray a nonstick frying pan with cooking spray. Heat over medium-high. Salt and pepper both sides of each breast half, place chicken breasts in pan, cover, reduce heat to simmer and cook, turning once, until done, approximately 7 minutes per side. About 4 minutes before done, spoon 1 tablespoon of orange-chipotle mixture on top of each breast. Cover and finish cooking. Remove from heat.

3 Place approximately ⅔ cup brown rice on each of 4 plates. Top with a chicken breast and the remaining orange-chipotle mixture.
Makes 4 servings.

Nutrition Analysis per serving: 409 calories, 5% fat (2.3 g; 0.6 g saturated), 66% carbs (67.5 g), 29% protein (29.7 g), 2.8 g fiber, 114 mg sodium

Kissed by an Italian Penne
(with the Touch of an Eggplant and Zucchini)

Directions

1 Bring pot of water to a boil and cook pasta according to directions on package or al dente. Rinse and set aside.

2 While pasta is cooking, spray a large, nonstick skillet with cooking spray and add oil. Heat over medium-high. Add onions and sauté, stirring occasionally, until translucent, approximately 5 minutes. Add garlic, eggplant and zucchini, and cook for 5 minutes, stirring occasionally. Add tomatoes, red pepper flakes, basil, Italian seasoning, tomato sauce, salt and pepper to taste. Stir to combine, cover and simmer for 10 minutes. Add spinach and toss. Cook for another 5 minutes. Remove from heat.

3 Place pasta on a large platter and top with sauce. Sprinkle with Parmesan and serve.
Makes 4 generous servings.

Ingredients

12 ounces uncooked whole-grain penne pasta

Cooking spray

1 tablespoon olive oil

2 cups diced yellow onion

1 tablespoon minced garlic

4 cups peeled and cubed eggplant

1 zucchini cut into ¾" cubes

1 ½ cups chopped Roma tomatoes

¼ teaspoon red pepper flakes

3 tablespoons chopped fresh basil leaves

1 teaspoon Italian seasoning

1 8-ounce can tomato sauce

Salt and pepper

2 cups baby spinach leaves

⅓ cup low-fat grated Parmesan cheese

Nutrition Analysis per serving: 425 calories, 14% fat (6.6 g; <1 g saturated), 71% carbs (75 g), 15% protein (16 g), 13.4 g fiber, 507 mg sodium

Bedded Herbed Salmon

Ingredients

Cooking spray

1 tablespoon fresh oregano leaves

1 tablespoon fresh rosemary

2 teaspoons fresh thyme leaves

1 tablespoon fresh parsley

1 tablespoon lemon peel

2 minced garlic cloves

¼ teaspoon fresh ground black pepper

½ cup bread crumbs

⅓ cup fat-free mayonnaise

Juice of 1 lemon

Salt to taste

1 ½ pounds wild Alaskan salmon fillet

1 tablespoon extra virgin olive oil

2 minced garlic cloves

2 tablespoons chicken broth

6 cups fresh baby spinach

Directions

Heat oven to 350°F. Coat baking sheet with cooking spray.

1 Blend oregano, rosemary, thyme, parsley, lemon peel and garlic in a food processor. Blend with pepper, bread crumbs, mayonnaise, lemon juice and salt in a small bowl until it forms clumps. Spread evenly on the salmon fillet. Place on cooking sheet and bake for 20–25 minutes or until salmon is almost done *(will be slightly translucent in center)*. Remove and cover to finish cooking.

2 In a medium, nonstick skillet, heat oil over medium heat. Add garlic and sauté for 5 minutes, add broth and spinach and sauté until spinach is wilted. Divide among 6 plates and top each with portion of salmon.
Makes 6 servings.

Nutrition Analysis: 285 calories, 47% fat (15 g; 3 g saturated), 17% carbs (12 g), 36% protein (26 g), 2 g fiber, 336 mg sodium

Orange-Scented Swiss Kisses

Directions

Place wax paper over a cookie sheet and coat with cooking spray.

1 In a double boiler over medium-high heat, place chocolate, cocoa powder, half & half and orange peel. Stir continuously until mixture is completely melted. Remove from heat.

2 Stir into chocolate mixture nuts, craisins and vanilla. Blend thoroughly.

3 Drop teaspoons of the chocolate-nut mixture onto wax paper–lined cookie sheet. Place in refrigerator to cool.
Makes 24 kisses.

Ingredients

Cooking spray

1 ¼ cups Swiss dark chocolate

2 tablespoons cocoa powder

1/4 cup fat-free half & half

1 tablespoon finely grated orange peel

1 cup chopped almonds and pecans

½ cup craisins

2 teaspoon vanilla extract

Nutrition Analysis per kiss: 88 calories, 51% fat (5 g; 1.8 g saturated), 41% carbs (9 g), 8% protein (1.8 g), 1.5 g fiber, 2 mg sodium

Is-That-a-Carrot-in-Your-Pocket-or-Are-You-Just-Glad-to-See-Me Cake

Ingredients

Cake:

1 ⅔ cups finely grated carrots

½ cup nonfat, plain yogurt

½ cup sugar

¼ cup Splenda

½ cup apple butter

¼ cup light olive oil

2 egg whites

1 ½ teaspoons cinnamon

¼ teaspoon ground cloves

¼ teaspoon nutmeg

Salt (optional)

1 teaspoon rum extract

1 cup dried tart cherries

¼ cup nonfat milk

1 ¼ cups whole-wheat flour

¾ cup unbleached, white flour

2 teaspoons baking soda

Frosting:

8 ounces fat-free cream cheese

¼ cup sugar

¼ cup Splenda

1 teaspoon rum extract

½ cup chopped walnuts

Directions

Heat oven to 325°F. Coat an 8" square baking dish with cooking spray.

1 Cake: In a large bowl, combine carrots, yogurt, sugar, Splenda, apple butter, oil, egg whites, cinnamon, cloves, nutmeg, salt *(if desired)*, extract, cherries and milk.

2 In a medium bowl, thoroughly mix flours and baking soda. Add to carrot mixture and blend until all ingredients are wet. Pour batter into coated pan and bake for 50 minutes, or until a toothpick inserted into the middle comes out clean. Remove from oven, let cool for 10 minutes, then remove from pan and finish cooling on a cake rack.

3 Frosting: In a small bowl, whip cream cheese, sugar, Splenda and extract until smooth. Fold in ¼ cup walnuts. Spread on the cake then sprinkle with remaining walnuts.

Makes 12 small servings.

Nutrition Analysis per serving: 271 calories, 26% fat (7.8 g; <1 g saturated), 63% carbs (42.7 g), 11% protein (7.5 g), 3.4 g fiber, 278 mg sodium

Rum-ba Crumble Love

Directions

Heat oven to 350°F. Coat 2-quart baking dish with cooking spray.

1 Crumble: In a medium bowl, combine oats, flours, nuts, sugar and spices. Set aside. In a small bowl, whip honey, oil and egg substitute. Set aside.

2 Filling: In a large nonstick frying pan, melt butter over medium-high heat. Add apples and sauté until tender but still firm, approximately 12 minutes, stirring frequently. Add cherries, cinnamon, allspice, extracts and ½ cup rum. Continue to sauté until liquid is thick, approximately 3 minutes. Remove from heat.

In a medium saucepan, combine brown sugar, Splenda and half & half, and cook over medium-high heat until sugar dissolves, approximately 2 minutes. Remove from heat.

In a small bowl, combine 3 tablespoons rum with cornstarch and whip until thoroughly mixed. Add to saucepan and blend. Add cornstarch mixture to apples and toss to thoroughly coat. Transfer to coated baking dish.

3 Add honey-oil mixture to flour-nut mixture and stir until barely moistened. Crumble into pieces and top apple mixture. Bake until golden and bubbly, approximately 30 minutes. Makes 12 servings.

Nutrition Analysis per serving: 278 calories, 27% fat (8.3 g; 1 g saturated), 64% carbs (44.5 g), 9% protein (6.3 g), 4.6 g fiber, 24 mg sodium

Ingredients

Cooking spray

Crumble:

¼ cup rolled oats

¼ cup unbleached flour

½ cup whole-wheat flour

½ cup chopped pecans

¼ cup chopped walnuts

¼ cup brown sugar

1 teaspoon cinnamon

¼ teaspoon allspice

3 tablespoons honey

2 tablespoons light olive oil

¼ cup liquid egg substitute

Filling:

1 tablespoon butter

3½ pounds Granny Smith apples, peeled, seeded and cut into ½" strips

⅔ cup dried tart cherries

1 teaspoon cinnamon

½ teaspoon allspice

1 teaspoon vanilla extract

1 teaspoon rum extract

½ cup plus 3 tablespoons dark rum

⅓ cup brown sugar

⅓ cup Splenda

3 tablespoons fat-free half & half

1 tablespoon cornstarch

Berry Quickie Ice Cream Pie

Ingredients

1 ½ cups graham cracker crumbs

1 tablespoon cocoa powder

3 tablespoons nonfat, plain yogurt

2 tablespoons brown sugar

2 tablespoons apple butter

1 ½-quarts slow-churned,
no sugar added vanilla ice cream

¼ cup fat-free
dark chocolate syrup

1 pound strawberries, washed,
dried, stemmed and cut in half

3 cups raspberries, washed
and dried

2 tablespoons sugar

1 tablespoon Splenda

2 tablespoons cornstarch

Directions

Heat oven to 350°F.

1 In a medium bowl, thoroughly blend crumbs, cocoa, yogurt, sugar and apple butter. Transfer to a deep-dish pie pan and pat evenly into bottom and sides. Bake for 7 minutes. Remove and cool.

2 Spoon ice cream into crust. Spread evenly and smooth top. Drizzle chocolate syrup in straight lines across the top, then draw the tip of a knife across the lines to form chevron patterns. Place in freezer until firm.

3 In a medium saucepan, place berries, sugar, Splenda and cornstarch. Toss to thoroughly cover berries then heat over medium-high until sauce clarifies and thickens. Remove and refrigerate.

4 To serve, cut pie into wedges, place on plates and top with berry topping.
Makes 12 servings.

Nutrition Analysis per serving: 220 calories, 19% fat (4.6 g; 2.4 g saturated), 72% carbs (39.6 g), 9% protein (5 g), 5 g fiber, 171 mg sodium

ACKNOWLEDGMENTS

A sincere and heartfelt thanks to all the amazing people in my life who not only contributed to the completion of this book, but are also the reason I am deeply grateful for life every single day. My dear friend and agent, David Smith, who has championed my causes and had my back for years. To my bike buddy, friend and editor, Deb Brody, who has walked arm and arm with me through so many books I've lost count. To Shara Alexander, the very best publicist in the whole world. To Wayne and Paisley, who over a platter of sushi and a bottle of wine helped me decide to write this book. To my clients, friends, coworkers and family members who took my advice and then were gracious enough to allow me to share their stories, trials and successes in this book. It is a blessing and an honor to have them in my life. To the researchers whose dedication and hard work provide the basis for the accurate and reliable information on which I have based my advice and career for the past 30 years. And, of course, I am so very thankful to my guardian angel(s) who brought the two best children in the whole world into my life, Lauren and Will. They have been a joy every single day and have allowed me to experience a richness and depth of love, commitment, loyalty and trust that I never would have known otherwise. I love you two with all my heart.

INDEX